WHY YOU SHOULD READ THIS BOOK

The Art of Spiritual Healing is the most complete book on healing you will ever read, or ever need. It is the ONLY book you will need for total health care — to heal your own self on higher levels, and to heal those around you. It contains comprehensive information on diet, nutrition, and spiritual healing on etheric levels.

Healing energy is *always* flowing through you. You will learn how to recognize and use this energy to remove blockages which cause disease and problems in your life.

Sherwood's style of writing is easy to read and straight forward. This book, *The Art of Spiritual Healing*, has already sold out of its first printing in the German edition. This American edition is presented in a no nonsense, down-to-earth, "hands on" approach. He has taken the mystery out of healing and has given us a very helpful "how to" book we can "lay our hands on".

The life saving contents of this book are so easy to understand, that after reading it, there is no reason why you could not become a successful healer and positively affect your own life and that of others you choose to work with — and they don't even have to be near you, or be aware of what you are doing, as you will learn in the chapter on Absentee Healing!

In a time when the *importance, necessity* and *value* of healthy living has become foremost in everyone's mind, and in a world *filled* with stressful situations, learn how to remove negativity and stress in a time proven step-by-step technique, and reprogram yourself to a optimum state of positive, healthful living.

Healing occurs on four planes. The highest is the spiritual plane, the residence of the "All", the Source of Healing. Next is the mental plane, which is the level of thought and mind. Then comes the etheric plane, the site of our emotions. Last is the physical plane, the level of physical matter, and the plane which most people erroneously believe is the only level of life, and where disease ultimately manifests itself.

Sherwood wants you to know that *you* can eliminate dis-ease and enjoy health and happiness, your rightful state of being.

About the Author

Keith Sherwood was born in New York in 1949. An internationally known teacher and healer, he founded the "American Psychic Association" and for two years was its director as well as editor of its magazine, *Psychic*. He has appeared on many radio and television shows in the United States and Europe. For three years he produced "Psychic Seminar," a weekly New York television program. He teaches "Chakra therapy," a synthesis of Western therapeutic techniques, Taoist Yoga and Tantra regularly throughout Europe.

His eclectic approach toward energy work is the outcome of years of study which took him first into psychotherapy as an encounter group therapist with New York City addicts. Later he traveled to the mountains of Guatemala where he studied with a Gurdieff master and trained in Yoga and Pranayama. He became a minister and worked in the Dominican Republic where his dormant powers as a healer and clairvoyant surfaced. After leaving the church in 1978 he devoted himself to the study of healing and human energy.

To Write to the Author

If you wish to contact the author or would like more information about this book, please write to the author in care of Llewellyn Worldwide, and we will forward your request. Both the author and publisher appreciate hearing from you and learning of your enjoyment of this book and how it has helped you. Llewellyn Worldwide cannot guarantee that every letter written to the author can be answered, but all will be forwarded. Please write to:

Keith Sherwood
c/o Llewellyn Worldwide
P.O. Box 64383-720, St. Paul, MN 55164-0383, U.S.A.

Please enclose a self-addressed, stamped envelope for reply, or $1.00 to cover costs.If outside the U.S.A., enclose international postal reply coupon.

Free Catalog from Llewellyn

For more than 90 years Llewellyn has brought its readers knowledge in the fields of metaphysics and human potential. Learn about the newest books in spiritual guidance, natural healing, astrology, occult philosophy and more. Enjoy book reviews, new age articles, a calendar of events, plus current advertised products and services. To get your free copy of *Llewellyn's New Worlds of Mind and Spirit*, send your name and address to:

Llewellyn's New Worlds of Mind and Spirit
P.O. Box 64383-720, St. Paul, MN 55164-0383, U.S.A.

ABOUT LLEWELLYN'S NEW AGE SERIES

The "New Age" — it's a phrase we use, but what does it mean? Does it mean the changing of the Zodiacal Tides, that we are entering the Aquarian Age? Does it mean that a new Messiah is coming to correct all that is wrong and make Earth into a Garden? Probably not — but the idea of a *major change* is there, combined with awareness that Earth *can* be a Garden; that war, crime, poverty, disease, etc., are not necessary "evils".

Optimists, dreamers, scientists . . . nearly all of us believe in a "better tomorrow", and that somehow we can do things now that will make for a better future life for ourselves and for coming generations.

In one sense, we all know "there's nothing new under the Heavens", and in another sense that "every day makes a new world". The difference is in our consciousness. And this is what the New Age is all about: it's a major change in consciousness found within each of us as we learn to bring forth and manifest "powers" that Humanity has always potentially had.

Evolution moves in "leaps". Individuals struggle to develop talents and powers, and their efforts build a "power bank" in the Collective Unconsciousness, the "soul" of Humanity that suddenly makes these same talents and powers easier access for the majority.

Those who talk about a New Age believe a new level of consciousness is becoming accessible that will allow anyone to manifest powers previously restricted to the few who had worked strenuously for them: powers such as Healing (for self and others), Creative Visualization, Psychic Perception, Out-of-Body Consciousness and more.

You still have to learn the 'rules' for developing and applying these powers, but it is more like a "relearning" than a *new* learning, because with the New Age it is as if the basis for these had become genetic.

The books in the New Age series are as much about ATTITUDE and AWARENESS as they are about the "mechanics" for learning and using Psychic, Mental, Spiritual, or Parapsychological Powers. Understanding that the Human Being is indeed a "potential god" is the first step towards the realization of that potential: expressing in outer life the inner creative powers.

Llewellyn's New Age Series

THE ART OF
SPIRITUAL HEALING

by
KEITH SHERWOOD

1994
Llewellyn Publications
St. Paul, Minnesota 55164-0383, U.S.A.

FIRST EDITION
Tenth Printing, 1994

Artwork by Michael Padgett

Library of Congress Cataloging-in-Publication Data
Sherwood, Keith.
    The art of spiritual healing / by Keith Sherwood. — St. Paul, Minn., U.S.A. : Llewellyn Publications, 1985.
    209 p.: ill.; 21 cm. — (Llewellyn's new age series)
    Bibliography: p. [201]-203.
    Includes index.
    ISBN 0-87542-720-0 (pbk.) : $7.95
    1. Spiritual healing. I. Title II. Series
BL65.M4S47   1985   615.8'52—dc19   85-10224

Llewellyn Publications
A Division of Llewellyn Worldwide, Ltd.
P.O. Box 64383, St. Paul, MN 55164-0383

TABLE OF CONTENTS

CHAPTER ONE

INTRODUCTION TO HEALING

Healing energy is *always* flowing through you. In this book you will learn how to recognize it and use it for healing yourself as well as those around you. It is my conviction that healing energy is available to everyone who is receptive to it, who believes it exists and expects it to transform one's life by changing disease into good health. It is a gift of God which is poured out to anyone who asks for it with an open heart. It can be likened to the renewing process which goes on continually in every healthy human being, and strives to keep everyone healthy all the time. The healer intercedes and helps accelerate the process of healing when good health has been disrupted; he acts as an agent to restore health, harmony and balance. It is called spiritual healing because God, the ALL, the source of healing, the Supreme Being, resides on the highest plane we can conceive of, the spiritual plane. From the spiritual plane, His essence is transmuted downward to the planes below.

In the *Bhagavad Gita* we read "the eternal spirit . . . everywhere are its hands and its feet, everywhere it has eyes that see, heads that think and mouths that speak: everywhere it listens; it dwells in all the worlds, it envelops them all."[1]

The Patient

In spiritual healing, the patient is not seen as the victim of disease. His behavior, attitude and lifestyle are viewed as important factors in promoting and nourishing the disease. As a result, the patient is always seen as the central protagonist in his own healing and is called upon to remain active rather than passive in spiritual healing. He is ultimately responsible for the healing of his own disease.

Spiritual healing, unlike other forms of healing (allopathic, homeopathic, chiropractic, etc.) relies on the ability of the healer to channel healing energy directly to his patient and the patient's ability to use that energy for one's own healing. This is largely an unconscious process that uses abilities which are dormant in all people. Medicine today seeks to alter the conditions in the human body so the body can heal itself, but it doesn't understand what healing is or where the energy for healing originates. Healing is far more than the removal of physical symptoms and the restoration of physical health; it is a return to balance and harmony. There can never be complete physical health unless the total being is healthy and in harmony with both its internal and external environments.

Total Health

Total health is the goal of spiritual healing.This goal is not something that is arrived at and then forgotten; healing is a process. We either move in the direction of health or in the direction of disease. It follows that each person must take individual responsibility for one's own health. There is never room for complacency when it comes to health because the human situation is never static. There are negative influences in our environment which push us towards disease, and there are positive influences which push us towards health. The healer pays attention to these influences and keeping them in mind, strives to alter negativity and replace it with what is positive. He or she seeks to heal on all levels.

The Healer

The healer's job is to identify the causes of disharmony and disease in the patient on whatever level they are found, and then to channel healing energy to the patient so the causes of the disease are eliminated, balance is restored and symptoms disappear. He accomplishes this by becoming a partner with the Divine will and allowing himself to be drawn into union with Divine consciousness. As he does this, he too, is healed by Divine energy, enriched by it and taught by it.

From the songs of Kabir we read: *tinwir sanjh ka gahira awai*

> The shadows of evening fall thick
>   and deep and the darkness of love
>   envelops the body and the mind.
> Open the window to the West, and be
>   lost in the sky of love;
> Drink the sweet honey that steeps
>   the petals of the lotus of the heart.
> Receive the waves in your body:
>   what splendour is in the region of the sea!
> Hark! the sounds of conches and bells are rising.
>
> Kabir says, "O brother, behold!
> The Lord is in this vessel of my body."[2]

As you might expect the healer has a unique view of health and disease. He doesn't see them in the same way as the average person. The healer doesn't see disease and health as separate conditions. In the same way he doesn't see life and death as separate conditions. The healer sees health and disease as opposite poles of the same thing, differing from each other in degree only. The healer understands those who are ill have allowed themselves to drift to the negative pole (disease) and now find it impossible to reach the opposite pole (good health) without outside help.

Disease
Disease is viewed as a swing to the negative pole which causes the disruption of good health throwing a per-

son out of balance. There is a direct link between the stress which disrupts good health and balance in a person's life, and the manifestation of physical symptoms. The stress caused by major disruptions in lifestyle have been studied and have been shown to have a major impact on health. Earlier this year, a report by the British medical journal *Lancet* cited that the incidence of fatal heart attacks increased markedly in Athens subsequent to the earthquake there in 1981. An Australian study of grief caused by the loss of a mate has shown that eight weeks after the spouse's death, the living partner has a weakened immunological system which makes him more vulnerable to negative influences in the environment, and thus more susceptible to disease. The American Academy of Family Physicians points out that two thirds of the office visits to physicians are prompted by stress related symtoms. Dr. Joel Elkes, director of the Behavioral Medicine Program at the University of Louisville tells us that the way we live and the way we conduct our lives is emerging as the most important cause of disease in America today.

Spiritual healers have always understood that disease is not caused solely by disease producing microbes. These creatures are not the root cause of disease. The illnesses they seem to cause are really symptoms of deeper problems due to imbalance which can usually be traced back to the higher planes.

Nourishment

There are four planes on which we humans live, and imbalance can originate on any of them. Imbalance is caused by separation, and a person can become separated from his source of nourishment on any of the four planes. Separation is most acute when it reaches the spiritual plane, when human beings become separated from the ALL, the source of spiritual nourishment. The Divine source eternally seeks union with its creation and could secure the health and harmony of each individual entity if the individual became consciously aware that he required spiritual nourishment to maintain good health. But this awareness is usually lacking, and consequently union is easily disrupted. When disruption occurs, the transfer of energy on the spiritual plane disrupts the transfer of healing energy from the ALL to the human spirit, and then there isn't sufficient energy available for transmutation to the lower planes. When this happens, an individual begins sliding towards the negative pole, the disease pole, and the renewing process which becomes weakened cannot neutralize negativity encountered on the lower planes.

The Four Planes

The healer sees the world as a living thing teeming with life on every level. He sees the universe as one large ecology of mind, body and spirit; all held in balance by God, the ALL.

He sees the universe as a complex system of interconnected levels vibrating at different frequencies. Different traditions have given different names to the various levels. To simplify things I will divide the universe into four distinct planes in accordance with the Western metaphysical tradition. This tradition is in large part derived from the ancient Hermetic philosophy and corresponds closely to Christian and Hindu teachings. The highest level is called the spiritual plane. It is the residence of the ALL, the healing source. Below the spiritual plane is the level of thought and mind which is called the mental plane. Next is the etheric plane, the site of our emotions. It is sometimes called the astral plane. Lastly, we come to the physical plane, which is the level of physical life and matter. Energy and matter of different vibrations exist on different planes. Energy of lower vibrations can be transmuted upward to the higher planes by having their vibrations increased, while higher vibrations may remain on the higher levels or may be transmuted from the higher levels for use on the lower ones. We humans straddle the dimensions, forming a bridge between the highest plane (spirit) and the lowest plane (matter).

Hermetics

Throughout this book, I will continue to refer to the Hermetic Philosophy and its importance in spiritual healing. Hermetics is the foundation, the bedrock on which our understanding of spiritual healing is built. An understanding of it is essential if the healer hopes to master the techniques of spiritual healing.

Hermetics originated in ancient Egypt. We are told that it was given to mankind by Thoth the Egyptian god of wisdom who the Greeks later called Hermes Trismegistrus. He was hailed from the earliest times as the "Master of Masters". If Hermes did exist, he is truly the father of esoteric wisdom. The details of his life have been lost to us, but one tradition has it that he was a contemporary of Abraham's. Perhaps he was the fabled Melchezidec, whom Abraham paid tithes to, or whom Jesus was compared to when he was described as "a priest on the order of Melchezidec."[3]

Whatever the truth may be, Hermes gave man a set of teachings which have influenced philosophy and religion ever since. His teachings are contained in a set of axioms which are set down for the modern student most succinctly in the *Kybalian*. From the *Kybalian*, we learn that the entire philosophy hinges on seven simple principles, and the practice of healing in its many forms is most clearly understood in Hermetic terms.

The first Hermetic Axiom states "The ALL is mind: the Universe is mental."[4] This doesn't mean what we see in the material world is an illusion, what the Hindus call *maya*. When the Hermeticist or healer says that everything is mental, he means that the source, the cosmic root of everything animate and inanimate is infinite creative mind. (verbalized in Sanskrit as OHM).

Human beings by being sentient and self-aware can experience infinite mind as it manifests in their spirit, through the I AM which is at the center of their being.

The second Hermetic Axiom states, "As above, so below; as below, so above." (the *Kybalian*). There are planes above us-higher dimensions-which would be beyond our understanding (hidden behind the veils) if the second Hermetic Axiom, the Principle of Correspondence didn't have universal application. Because the Principle of Correspondence applies to all levels at all times, man can begin to understand the higher planes by studying the lower ones.

The third Hermetic Axiom, the Principle of Vibration states that "nothing rests; everything moves; everything vibrates."[6]

Applying the Principle of Vibration to healing, we can see that not only does everything vibrate, but everything that vibrates has a characteristic rate of vibration which is its unique mark. This vibration can be influenced negatively or positively by other vibrations in the environment. When a person's vibration is negatively affected, disease results. The process of healing is the process of correcting a person's rate of vibration. We can illustrate this by thinking of disease as a wobble or an unrhythmic vibration. In a car when the tires are poorly aligned, a wobble develops which affects the steering; to correct it, a person must have the alignment checked and then have the wheels balanced. Once the wobble develops, its uncharacteristic vibration can adversely affect other systems in the car; the same thing can occur in the human system. Disease in one area can create disease in a related area or in a nearby system. A wobble also can begin on one level and can be transmuted to the level adjacent to it. For example, an unrhythmic vibration on the etheric plane if not corrected will damage both the mental plane and the physical plane.

The fourth Hermetic Axiom is called the Principle of Polarity. It states that "everything is dual; everything has poles; everything has its pair of opposites; like and unlike are the same; opposites are identical in nature, but different in degree; extremes meet; all truths are but half truths; all paradoxes may be reconciled."[7] From this principle we can deduce that spirit and matter are simply two poles of the same thing, and everything between them has elements of both, varying from each other only in degree (i.e. vibration). If opposites are really the same and if spirit and matter are the same thing (differing only in their rate of vibration), then they are transmutable, and spiritual energy can positively affect anything in the physical world, including the physical body. It follows in the human experience that hate can be transmuted into love; pain into joy; disease into perfect health. Because the healer understands the Principle of Polarity, he can transmute negative energy into positive energy on every level.

The fifth Hermetic Axiom states that "everything flows out and in; everything has its tides; all things rise and fall; the pendulum swing manifests in everything; the measure of the swing to the right is the measure of the swing to the left; rhythm compensates."[8]

The healer understands the law of rhythm and becomes attentive, and "pays attention" to the natural rhythm he finds everywhere, especially those within himself. He learns that rhythm compensates and like the great physician Hippocrates said,"Opposites are cures for opposites."[9]

By becoming attentive to his own rhythms and his patient's rhythms, the healer can see the "wobble" in any particular rhythm and can transmute healing energy into the exact vibration or dosage which will compensate for the disease or wobble he finds in his patient.

The sixth Hermetic Axiom states that "every cause has its effect; every effect has its cause; everything happens according to the law; chance is but a name for law not recognized; there are many planes of causation, but nothing escapes the law."[10] The most important feature of this Principle of Healing is that nothing happens by chance; the root of every disease is a chain of events which the ill person participated in, even if his participation was largely unconscious. In the final tally he is responsible, and as a result he will eventually pay the price for past actions through present disease and pain. This law of cause and effect is called *karma*. In the book of Galatians the Apostle Paul tells us," . . .God is not mocked, for whatever a man soweth, that he shall also reap."[1] [1]

The seventh Hermetic Axiom is the Principle of Gender. It states that "gender is in everything; everything has its masculine and feminine principles; gender manifests on all planes."[1] [2] Gender, it should be understood, represents far more than sex; the differences between male and female which are quite clear to us on the physical plane. Gender manifests on all planes. On the mental plane, the masculine principle of gender is manifest as the objective mind, the conscious active mind. The feminine aspect corresponds to the subjective, unconscious passive mind. On the emotional plane, the masculine principle manifests itself as assertiveness, anger and all extroverted emotions. The feminine principle manifests itself as receptivity, protection, and all introverted emotions. This duality is inherent in all living things, including human beings. As human beings, we have within us the masculine assertive element and the feminine receptive element. It is the healer's job to integrate this dual nature first within himself. and then within his patient; to bring everyone he works with into harmony and balance.

CHAPTER TWO

THE DANGER OF FEAR

It is our state of mind more than anything else which determines how healthy we will be. Thus, in spiritual healing, we begin counteracting disease by interceding on the mental plane, the most accessible level to us.

Most of us have a personal code, a belief system which guides our lives, and our belief system is largely determined by our environment and what we have experienced and learned from it. Our schools, families, friends, the books we have read all influence us. They have helped to mold us into who we are today. People and institutions have helped to shape our view of the universe, programming us and influencing how we see ourselves, how healthy we will be, how we react, what we want and even what we fear. The Bible speaks at length about the danger of inordinate fear. In the Old Testament Isaiah tells us, "Sanctify the Lord of hosts himself: and let him be your fear, and let him be your dread, and he shall be for a sanctuary . . ."[13] and later, in the New Testament, we are told "For God has not given us that spirit of fear but of power and of love, and of a sound mind."[14] It is the spirit of fear and its sidekicks: anxiety, doubt and worry which are the greatest threats to good health.

Although our fears are often subjective and groundless, our unconscious mind is childlike; it believes what the conscious mind tells it, and it cannot differentiate between fact and fiction. And so the unconscious mind will be tormented

11

by phantoms and monsters if negative programming in the form of negative thoughts and imagination is allowed free reign in the conscious mind. When a person is governed by a belief system which promotes fear; unreal thoughts become real things, and when this happens a person can become victimized by worries and anxieties that have no basis in reality but which later can produce physical disease. The following story illustrates the effects of negative imagination:

> A somewhat inebriated gentleman was slowly moving along the street, carrying in his hands a box with perforations in the lid and sides. It appeared he was carrying some live animal in the box. An acquaintance stopped him and asked, "What have you got in the box?"
> "It is a mongoose," replied the tipsy man.
> "What on earth for?"
> "Well, you know how it is with me; I am not really drunk now, but I soon shall be. And when I am, I see snakes all around and I get awfully scared. That is what I got the mongoose for; to protect me from the snakes!"
> "Good heavens, those are imaginary snakes!"
> "This also is an imaginary mongoose!"
> The box was, in fact, empty.[15]

This story, although amusing, shows us that the mind must be purged of negativity and brought under control if a person hopes to regain inner harmony and freedom from negative imagination and disease.

Dr. Caroline Thomas has studied the long-term health records of 1,337 medical students from 1948 to 1964 and has found that negative feelings towards one's family can be a leading indicator for those who in later life developed cancer, mental illness or committed suicide. Dr. Carl Simington tells us " . . . it seems logical that if a person is able to mentally influence whether or not the disease (cancer) spreads or is able to gain control of his disease, it only makes sense that he has something to do with developing the disease in the first place."[16]

Negative Programming

Since thought precedes action, it follows that if you imagine yourself to be a certain "kind" of person, your actions will be predetermined by your imagination. Moreover, if your behavior is influenced by what people say about you, then your behavior will be programmed by the people around you. Thus, your personal reality, no matter how complex, will be determined not by you but by your conditioning.

If over the years you have been programmed negatively in any area of your life by family, friends and institutions, then you have suffered until now from their negativity. Also, you will continue to suffer, perhaps more heavily in the future as negativity takes its toll on your physical body. Negative programming on any level has an insidious effect on the physical body, slowly breaking it down; eroding good health little by little over the years. We can see the dramatic effects of negativity on children in psychologically related diseases, but these constitute only the tip of the iceberg. Negativity is the unseen agent of disease for every member of the human race. It affects all of us, especially those who are most sensitive.

All your life you have been programmed to behave in certain ways, to accept certain beliefs and to live by certain rules. You have developed a belief system which influences you in your career, relationships and health. Your belief system, created by this programming and your reaction to it determines how you will live. It is not always the most effecient and satisfying system to follow, however, since it can bring you into conflict with your own natural urges, desires and needs. Programming of this kind, by being disruptive, can knock you off balance, create disharmony and cause wear and tear on your physical body. It can be a time bomb which makes the development of disease inevitable because of the restriction and stress it causes. But you needn't be slavishly controlled or physically damaged by negative programming. As you will see in later chapters, the effect of negative programming can be reversed and the negative programming itself can be replaced with positive programming, which will nourish you and provide the structure for good health and happiness.

Overcoming Negativity

You can transcend the limitations imposed upon you by negative programming and a restrictive belief system and like healers and shamans, metaphysicians and alchemists, holy men and women, who have sought ways to open themselves to the Divine healing force, you can become a channel for healing. You can alter your lifestyle and take total responsibility for your life, your health and well-being. You can learn to overcome stress, to resist negative programming on any level. You can learn to open your inner channels so that you can be healed. You can open yourself and allow the I AM (your higher self) to emerge and you can become whole again. This has been my quest. As a healer, I will share with you what I have learned and explain how I succeeded in opening the channels within me and how I focus the healing energy which inevitably comes through. I will share with you what I've learned from my teachers and from the ancients, whose work remains extant. You will learn the most practical techniques available and use them as a guide for your own spiritual development. As you progress you will come into Union with the healing force which is a direct manifestation of God, the ALL, and it will lead each of you into a deeper understanding of who you really are. A person who has transcended negativity has come back into balance and has opened a channel for the healing force to flow. He who has learned to become whole again can accomplish remarkable things, as we can learn from the Second Book of Kings:

And the woman conceived, and bore a son at the season that Elisha had said unto her, according to the set time. And when the child was grown, it fell on a day that he went out to his father to the reapers. And he said unto his father, "My head, my head." And he said to a lad, "Carry him to his mother." And when he had taken him, and brought him to his mother, he sat on her knees till noon. And she went up, and laid him on the bed of the man of God, and shut the door upon him, and went out . . . And when Elisha was come into the house, behold, the child was dead, and lay upon his bed. He went in, therefore, and shut the door upon the two of them, and prayed unto the Lord. And he went up, and lay upon the child, and put his mouth upon his mouth, and his eyes upon his eyes, and his hands upon his hands: and he stretched himself upon the child; and the flesh of the child became warm. Then he returned, and walked in the house to and fro, and went up, and stretched himself upon him; and the child sneezed seven times, and the child opened his eyes. And he called Gehazi, and said, "Call this Shunammite." So he called her. And when she was come in unto him, he said, "Take up thy son."[17]

Opening Up

Those of you who practice healing will be stretched to the limits of your creativity. The healer, by becoming a tool of the Divine will (a channel of healing energy) transcends the finite and becomes a conduit for infinite love and power. During the act of healing, the healer transcends human limitation, the I AM emerges, and with God becomes a participant in a Divine dance, truly a dance of life! God has no favorites and His gifts are poured out to all those who sincerely need and desire them. Those of you who have a sincere desire to be a channel, to be a healer, to be healed, and to heal others will not be disappointed. You must follow your desire to be of service and to heal. Your desire is your key. Use it to open your inner doors through which God's healing power will flow. Remember that if you ask God for bread, he won't give you a stone, but *manna*, spiritual bread, the bread of life which you must then share with everyone else who hungers for it. Healing is the bread of life, because healing is the process of renewing life.

To open yourselves and to become channels you must begin by learning to "pay attention", then you must "re-member" who you are and "recollect" your "self." The purpose of this book is to teach you to "pay attention" and guide you into "remembrance and recollection", which will bring you back into "relationship" and finally into union with your source of nourishment, the ALL, so that you can live in perfect health and become a channel for healing, serving those who suffer from disease of any kind. The Buddhist would insist that you've always been in union with the ALL, but that in your ignorance you have forgotten that you are. I must agree, but would also add that not only are you in union with the ALL, but you are a channel for healing as well. In spiritual healing, you must begin by remembering that as a child you already were a channel but as you grew older, you stopped paying attention. The channels were neglected, fell into disrepair and were forgotten. But now, by paying attention again, you can remember who you are and by opening yourself you can become a channel for healing. The Divine healing force is given freely to all who ask. All that is necessary is that the way be opened for it.

You must clean out those clogged channels and bring them back into service; the service of a world desperately in need of healing.

The opening of our inner channels is essentially what healing is about. When the Divine healing power floods your being, you can be healed. When this same spiritual energy or *prana* as it is called in Sanskrit is focused towards another person, then you act as a channel for his healing. It is the process of transmuting energy. Energy coming from the spiritual plane enters your spirit and is transmuted. It then enters your mind (the mental plane); next, your emotions (the etheric plane); and from there it flows into your physical body. This process is a natural one which takes place all the time in healthy human beings.

The Healer's Tools

I will be dividing the subject matter of this book into three parts: diagnosis, absentee healing and "laying on of hands". You will learn how to diagnose disease in your patients. You will learn to see auras and to diagnose from them as well as to feel the aura and diagnose problems in your patient's "subtle energy system". You will learn techniques designed to reawaken your dormant psychic powers so that you can clairvoyantly "see" and clairsentiently "feel" the physical ailments in your patients. I will teach you how to channel healing energy from a distance. I call this absentee healing. It is sometimes called mental healing, but mental healing leaves it incomplete. Even at a distance, the healer can project more than healing thoughts; he can send healing rays and he can use color to heal. Furthermore, the healer can project his consciousness within his patient's body and work directly on the diseased area. In absentee healing, you will learn to function in deeper levels of consciousness, and from these levels you will learn to project rays of energy from your *chakras* (energy centers); you will also learn to use verbal affirmations and visualizations to heal.

In the laying on of hands, you will learn to heal through vibration; through polarization; and finally, through empathetic healing, a process which will bring you into union with your patient. I will lead you through meditations and techniques designed to open and balance your chakras. You will learn to relax completely and breathe properly so that you can channel greater quantities of *prana* (healing energy) into and through your body. Not only will this book teach you the techniques necessary for healing others, but you will also learn how to heal yourself.

CHAPTER THREE

THE HEALER WITHIN

To understand disease, health and how the healer can transmute disease into good health, you must understand that you are far more than you think you are; whatever your limitations, they are self-imposed. Dr. Frederic Tilney, one of France's foremost brain specialists, has stated that in the future, "We will, by conscious demand, evolve cerebral centers which will permit us to use (mental) powers that we now are not even capable of imagining."[18]

The concept of increased human potential is nothing new. If we go back two thousand years, we learn that Jesus told His disciples, "If ye have faith as a grain of mustard seed, ye shall say unto this mountain, Remove hence to yonder place; and it shall remove; and nothing shall be impossible to you."[19] The extraordinary potential and power which lies dormant within each of us is a manifestation of the unconscious self, what is often called the I AM. It is just below the surface, below consciousness. It is from this inner reservoir that our extraordinary powers spring. Healing is one of these powers.

The *Bhagavad Gita* tells us, "Though the saint sees, hears, touches, smells, eats, moves, sleeps, breathes, yet he knows the truth and he knows that it is not he who acts.[20] The healer knows that the conscious self is not the healer. He knows that it is never the lower self or ego who heals. At best, the lower self gives permission and moves aside for the unconscious self, the I AM to act. To move

19

the conscious self aside, you must begin by "paying attention". Only then will you see the unconscious for what it is. You will discover that it is not monolithic; it has a complex character which will seem both familiar and alien to you as you begin to uncover its qualities. My description of the unconscious self and the planes on which it functions will be merely an outline.

I will give you only the most salient features and as you progress, you can fill in the details as you uncover them. The unconscious self and the inner environment of each person is subjective, unique in many ways, and for each person the particular details differ. Each human being is a synthesis of conscious and unconscious elements. The conscious self is associated with the physical world. The unconscious self is concerned with the non physical worlds or higher vibration.

The Four Bodies

Our universe is composed of four planes or dimensions, and each human being is composed of four bodies which exist on these planes. On the conscious level, we have a physical body which dwells on the physical plane. The physical body gives and receives information through the five senses and receives its nourishment through the food, water and air it breathes. It is composed of dense matter vibrating at a low frequency. It is through the physical body that the true being, which is the unconscious self, experiences the physical world. The physical world is made up of what we call matter, and the energies and forces which cause matter to react.

You must remember these divisions are somewhat arbitrary since nothing has a separate existence outside the All. The divisions or planes, and our separate bodies are being classified here for convenience's sake. The physical body as understood by the healer is not considered a thing separate in itself; in the same way that he doesn't consider matter as a unique substance. He sees matter as energy, albeit of a lower vibration. In the same way he sees the physical body as a manifestation of the All, but of a lower vibration.

This conforms to the Hermetic Principle of Correspondence, which teaches us that, "As above, so below".[21] Applying this principle of correspondence to spiritual healing, you can see the physical health of any human being is directly related to the health of his higher bodies, which vibrate at higher frequencies.

The Etheric Body

Each of us has within the physical body an etheric body, which for the most part conforms to the size and shape of its physical counterpart. The etheric body, like the physical body, is an actual body made up of material, although it vibrates at a much faster frequency than physical matter. You can conceive of its position in relation to the physical body by using the analogy of a Russian doll. It fits into the physical body like a hand fits into a glove.

The principle of "interpenetration" which we must address next, explains that the astral or etheric plane is a condition rather than a locality; as every physical atom, molecule and body floats in a sea of astral matter. Astral matter interpenetrates physical matter and your astral body interpenetrates your physical body.

The astral body's main function is to provide the physical body with the energy it needs to remain sentient and to keep it connected to the energy web which underlies the universe. It does this through what I call the "subtle energy system" which is composed of: the *chakras* — the seven major energy centers found along the spine (see plate); the minor energy centers scattered throughout the body; the meridians which connect them; as well as the aura which surrounds the physical body and forms a protective egg shaped shield around it. It is through the chakras located on the surface of the etheric body that energy enters the physical body from the higher planes. Alice Bailey in her exhaustive work *Esoteric Healing* explains, "The etheric body is fundamentally the most

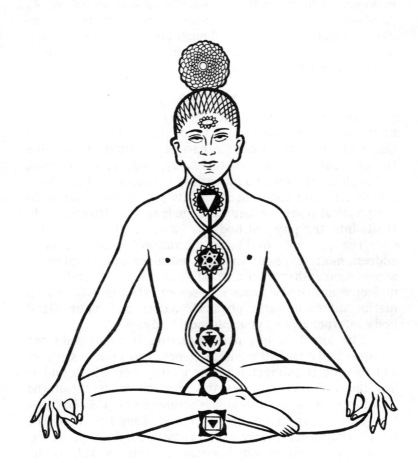

Plate 1: The Seven Chakras

important response apparatus which man possesses, producing not only the right functioning of the five senses and consequently providing five major points of contact with the tangible world, but it also enables man to register sensitively the subtler worlds . . ."[22]

The Mental Body

Interpenetrating both the etheric body and the physical body is the mental body. It is the center of thought and along with the etheric body constitutes what is often called the soul. It receives and transmits thoughts from other sentient creatures as well as receiving thoughts from the All as they are transmuted from the spiritual to the mental plane. This process of transmutation explains how new ideas enter the finite human mind from the infinite mind of the All. At the appropriate times, God provides receptive minds with new and innovative ideas. In healing, we give great importance to the mental body since many of our maladies originate there. In time the disorders are transmuted to the etheric body, causing inordinate desire, negative moods, lack of vitality, overindulgence, etc. Negative thoughts that originate in other people's minds can be transferred to the unwary mind if the mental aura which shields the healthy mind is weakened. And, the adoption of a negative belief system in childhood can undermine the health of the mental body unless a person learns how to filter out negative thoughts and replace them with positive ones.

The soul, which is composed of the etheric body and the mental body, can be influenced by both the spiritual body and its desires. The physical body and its desire and the course of a person's life and health is largely determined by how one integrates the forces acting on one's "individual soul".

The Spiritual Body

The spiritual body is the body of highest vibration. It dwells on the spiritual plane, which is the site of infinite mind, the All.

From the spiritual plane, the most radiant and profound energy enters a human being's spiritual body. From
there it is transmuted so that it can be used on the lower
planes. The human spirit is not a separate body like the
mental, etheric or physical body. It is a direct manifestation of the All and as such is a synthesis of God and man.

If a person's spiritual connection with the All is weakened, so is his spiritual body, because it is cut off from its
source of spiritual nourishment which is infinite mind.
When a person is unaware of his spiritual nature and his
need for spiritual sustenance, he can inadvertently encourage the development of disease in the spiritual body. Disease
in the spiritual body will sooner or later be transmuted
downwards until it infects the physical body.

Edgar Cayce was once asked about the importance of
spiritual energy in healing. He stated while in trance,
"Through trust in spiritual things, the quicker will be the
response in the physical body. For all healing—mental and
material—is attuning each atom of the body, each reflex of
the brain, to awareness of the Divine that lies within each
atom, each cell."[23]

It is from the spiritual plane (the level of infinite mind
as opposed to finite mind) that the All, God, became and
continues to become transmuted, allowing His infinite
nature to flow into the level of mind and becoming manifest there as finite mind and as thought. The process continues as thought is transmuted to the lower planes by
having its vibration lowered.

Plato understood this process when he spoke of
"forms", explaining that behind every material object is
a pure "thought form". So did the Apostle John, when
he described Christ as the "Word" (God's thought made
manifest), explaining that: "In the beginning was the Word
and the Word was with God, and the Word was God . . .
All things were made by Him; and without Him was not
anything made that was made."[24]

Paying Attention

Only by "paying attention" can a person become aware of his complex nature and his relationship with God. Paying attention is a way of life for the healer. It is a different form of perception than normal cognition. Learning to pay attention is essential in spiritual healing, but it is not a simple task. Although paying attention may begin as an act of will, will power alone is incapable of keeping a person's attention on an object or person for long. If you attempt to pay attention to an object with your will power alone, you will notice after a short time your attention drifts; it is swayed by some passing thought or feeling. You will find that even with the best intentions it is difficult to keep your mind from roving to and fro.

Although it might be difficult to pay attention at first, with practice you will find it soon becomes quite easy and more satisfying than your normal means of experiencing the world.

Paying attention is the starting point in the practice of spiritual healing. Paying attention is important in healing, but it should not be confused with concentration. Concentration, as most people understand it, is a purely mental process in which an individual directs his attention exclusively to one object and closes himself off to everything else. There are some methods of meditation which are concentrative methods, but I have found that concentration has little value in healing because it is solely a mental process.

What you need in healing is a way to pay attention to one thing, not concentrating on it. I have found this cannot be done by pushing everything out of the way and then, by an act of will, force the mind to stay on one thing. Paying attention, unlike concentration, requires the cooperation of the mind and heart. Rather than pushing things out of the way as they enter the conscious mind, you need only look at something first with your conscious mind. Then if you open your heart to it and hold it with the attention of your unconscious mind with love and compassion, and it will not waver. While you are paying attention you can allow the conscious mind the freedom to wander where it likes. The unconscious mind, which is directly connected with your heart center will keep the object in focus as long as your heart is centered on it. Paying attention is a manifestation of the feminine, receptive aspect of human nature as outlined in the seventh Hermetic Axiom, the Principle of Gender.

By paying attention, the healer learns to relate to the world with heart and mind in balance. There is cooperation between the masculine, assertive elements and the feminine, receptive aspects (conscious mind and unconscious mind or heart).

Moreover, paying attention doesn't involve analysis or comparison. In analysis, the observer does more than become visually aware of something in the environment; he seeks to understand what he sees in terms of his past experience. He alters what he sees by subjectively passing the experience through a mental filter.

In paying attention, you must abstain from subjectifying the experience by detaching yourself from what you perceive through your senses. You see without participating (you see objectively).

Even in a court of law, it is recognized that prior prejudice will alter a witness' perception of events or a juror's objectivity in determining the truth of what he or she has experienced.

Paying attention may begin as act of will, but it comes to fruition as an act of surrender. This is achieved when you open your heart to the object of your attention and become receptive to it. Rather than imposing your will on the environment, you learn to put your will into the service of the All, and then you begin to see things as they really are; not as you would like them to be.

Seeing reality, seeing things as they really are, however, is nothing new . . .

It is a return to the natural human condition which you experienced as a child. It becomes possible only after the feminine aspect of your nature (which is associated with the heart and unconscious mind) becomes integrated with the masculine assertive aspect and you become receptive to the energy which flows through you from God, the All, as He manifests on the different planes. Paying attention, surrender and the suspension of analysis and judgement—at least momentarily—are essential in healing and in experiencing things as they really are.

Most of you have forgotten what the childlike condition was like. In healing, however, remembering it is very important. In the Bible we read, "Whosoever shall not receive the kingdom of God like a little child shall in no way enter it."[25] We read in the Tao, "Without stirring abroad, one can know the whole world; without looking out the window, one can see the way of heaven. The further one goes, the less one knows. Therefore, the sage knows, without having to stir, identifies without having to see, accomplishes without having to act."[26] The healer, like the sage, pays attention. He sees the world as it is and in the process remembers who he is; he stops trying to alter things and becomes receptive instead.

Remembrance and Recollection

Returning to the way, the Tao, is what I call remembrance. Remembrance is experiencing yourself as you are and the Universe as it really is. You experience yourself in your proper role and in your proper *Dharma* (life path). By paying attention you see reality and how you fit into it.

P. D. Ouspensky tell us that, "To remember one's self means the same thing as to be aware of one's self—I AM. Sometimes it comes by itself; it is a very strange feeling. It is not a function; not thinking, not feeling; it is a different state of consciousness."[27] Remembrance revives the knowledge that we exist on more than one level and by nature we are polar, containing both masculine and feminine elements on all levels regardless of physical gender, being both assertive and receptive.

Once you've learned the Universe is more than mundane, gross material existence and once you have started to integrate your conscious and unconscious selves, you will begin to experience the reality of who you are, and you will see that you are not just a physical being. You are not confined to experiencing the world through your senses alone. Each of you is a multidimensional being functioning simultaneously on all planes.

Like the All, you express yourself on every dimension, influencing and being influenced on every dimension. If you can pay attention and remember this, you can recollect yourself, put yourself together and become whole again. Integrating your four natures; spiritual, mental, emotional and physical, is what I mean by recollecting. By experiencing yourself as you exist on all levels, you can learn to consciously tap the sources of energy from even the highest plane, the spiritual plane, and then use these energies from all planes for healing.

Relationship and Love

Remembrance and recollection bring you into relationship with your source of nourishment; you learn to become receptive to what is positive and nourishing and you learn to resist what is negative and destructive on each plane.

Relationship on any plane can lead you into union, but relationship and finally union necessitate two parties. As a result, if you desire relationship, love is essential. The Principle of Correspondence teaches that you can make inferences about love on the higher planes by studying love on the physical and etheric planes.

You will see as we proceed that relationship and love in their highest forms are essential ingredients in healing. When I speak of love, I refer to the force which prompts a person to seek relationship with someone or something. In English, we have one word for that force, but in Greek there are three. The three words for love are *eros*, or sexual physical love; *filio*, brotherly love; and finally *agape*, divine love. These three terms describe conditions of human affection. When a person feels affection, he normally reacts by seeking relationship with the object of his affection, to make closer contact, to experience the object more deeply and usually to extend the duration of the experience. In other words, the act of loving in any form causes one to move towards the object of that love. Once a person attains the object of his or her love, he or she can have different experiences because the three kinds of love manifest different vibrations. When a person unites with the object of one's sexual love (eros), this produces a physical relationship and a physical gratification. By itself, it is a temporary relationship and it causes a person to seek gratification over and over again; because sexual satisfaction by its very nature is temporary. When a person seeks relationship on the higher planes, when he seeks agape love (spiritual relationship), the results are strikingly different. That is because the vibration of agape love, a form of selfless love which can only come from the spiritual plane, is higher than erotic love. The higher the vibration, the more permanent and deeper becomes the experience of relationship. Thus, agape love produces a permanent satisfaction or fulfillment which leads to union, while eros and filio (brotherly love) by their nature cannot. The added ingredient in agape love which makes union possible is God's grace which can only be extended to those who have faith in Him.

Faith and Union

It is the relationship formed through the lower vibrations which eventually leads the healer into relationship on the higher planes with God and with his patients. The healer learns about agape love by channeling human love (filio); human love becomes his teacher and the inner doorways open, permitting agape love to flow through him, if he has the faith to sustain it; and into the patient, if his patient has the faith to accept it. The healer reaches out in two directions, first to God, achieving relationship with the All, the source of healing, and then with his patient, becoming a channel between them through which the heal-

ing energy flows. The vibrations experienced in relationship
may be different, depending on what one has a relationship
with. But, it is from relationship on the lower dimensions
that one learns to surrender; and from the experience of
surrender, a person learns to raise his vibration. Moreover,
when a person reaches the necessary vibration through
agape love and faith, he becomes permanently united with
the source of healing, the All, who is spirit. Then the energy of the All can flow continually through him into his
patients, then into the environment. As we can see, the
healer should begin by achieving relationship with his
patient on the lower planes (lower vibrations), but he
should always strive to achieve union on the highest plane
as well.

The Bible tells us that faith, " . . . is the substance of
things hoped for, the evidence of things not seen.[28] and
then goes on to say, " . . . without faith it is impossible to
please Him (God); for he that cometh to God must believe
that He is, and that He is a rewarder of them that diligently
seek Him."[29] Love brings us into relationship with God,
the All, the healing source from whom spiritual nourishment comes, but faith keeps us in relationship and brings
us into union.

Faith is almost impossible to define but I agree with
most authorities that faith is, more than anything else, a
gift. From the spiritual plane the author of faith is the All,
God. With faith, like love, there is the elevation of the soul
from the lower planes to the higher planes; from the finite
to the infinite. But unlike love, faith is a state which is solely
the result of being grasped by the power of "being" which
transcends everything. Faith cannot be manufactured and
it cannot be understood in terms of anything else. It can
be imparted to us only by the All, God Himself. Faith is
never a state that a person has or has evolved to; it is a state
of divinity within the individual which affirms to that person he is unconditionally accepted and is part of the All. It
goes beyond relationship, which involves two consenting
parties, and retains the element of duality. On the human

side, relationship can be strained or severed temporarily by a change of mood, belief, etc. But with faith, duality is abolished as is separation, because in faith, God reaches out and brings a person unto Himself.

Once separation is abolished and nourishment is permanently established, those who have attained union become God's agents to nourish and heal the world; to lead those open and willing into relationship with God so they can be permanently reunited through the gift of faith.

CHAPTER FOUR

MENTAL DISEASE

"Mind is ever the builder. That which the body-mind feeds upon is what it gradually becomes."[30]

The mind can be likened to an arena where conflicting forces confront each other. On one side are arrayed positive thoughts and attitudes which produce good effects and therefore help maintain good health in the physical body; and on the other side are negative thoughts and attitudes which produce negative effects and in time negatively affect the physical body.

The mental influence on disease has received a great deal of attention in the past three decades and the investigator can now find a wealth of information in this area. Several long-term studies have shown that personality and attitude play a significant role in the development and progress of disease. In the case of cancer, the mental factor influences the susceptibility and treatment of the disease. Research indicates those people with negative attitudes, mental habits and ideas are far more susceptible to cancer, (this rule applies to other diseases as well) and they do far worse in treatment than those whose personalities differ. The most negative aspects of the cancer personality seem to be a tendency towards self-pity, which goes hand in hand with a very poor self-image. The cancer patient often has an underdeveloped capacity to trust either himself or others, which can be traced to early childhood rejection. The cancer patient has a strong tendency to hold anger in and to harbor

33

resentment. Because of his inability to forgive and forget and his lack of trust, the cancer patient often finds it difficult to develop and maintain long-term intimate relationships.

Affirmations and Visualizations

Healers have always understood that a negative mental state is the breeding ground for disease. Therefore, healers begin by counteracting disease on the mental plane by using affirmations and visualizations. These are two of the healer's most powerful tools. To be effective, the healer must understand how the human mind works; his healing strategy must be based on an accurate estimation of his patient's situation and mental state. The mental body must be healed as well as the physical body if the patient is to regain harmony and be freed from disease on the physical plane. The healer knows this can only be done if attitudes are changed and positive imagination is substituted for negative imagination whenever and wherever it is encountered; otherwise the patient will be tossed about not only by his own negative imagination, but also by the thoughts and imaginations of the people around him. Thoughts are real. They can be transferred through the ether from one mind to another; negative thoughts generated from one mind can be harmful to someone else. We are told in the book of Proverbs: "Make no friendship with an angry man . . . lest thou learn his ways"[31] This is not an idle warning!

There are many types of negative thoughts, but regardless of the endless varieties, all negative thoughts stem from frustrated desire and fear. Since desire and fear are forever subjective, they never accurately describe objective reality on the physical plane or any other plane.

Changing negative thought patterns into positive ones is the first order of business in healing yourself and healing others. It is called mental transmutation. In the Hermetic philosophy, it is stated this way: "Mind may be transmuted from state to state; degree to degree; condition to condition; pole to pole; vibration to vibration."[32] Transmuta-

tion is most easily understood if you think of it as reprogramming. All your life you have been programmed by
your environment and people around you. If you understand the concept of mental transmutation, you can learn
to change yourself by changing the way you think. Negativity subverts you from inside and attacks you from the
outside. Negativity usually strikes you first on the mental
plane. If it is not stopped there it is very rapidly transmuted to the etheric plane where it produces negative feelings
and an emotional contraction. Then your physical body
reacts by becoming anxious. Your muscles contract, your
breathing becomes shallow, etc. Willpower alone usually
can't help you overcome negativity and for a good reason.
Negative thoughts conjure up negative imagination and
negative imagination causes negative feelings. When the will
and the imagination are in conflict, it is always the imagination which wins. Emile Coue, the great French metaphy-
sician wrote, "Our actions spring not from our will, but
from our imagination."[33]

    Negative thoughts are transmitted verbally and visual-
ly. When negative verbal thoughts disturb you, you must
use words to transmute their negative effect. In Tibet the
monks say, "Neti, neti", (not this, not this) when they
want to remove negative thoughts from their mind. I prefer
to use "Cancel, cancel", the technique developed by Jose
Silva. Once you begin paying attention to your thoughts,
you will be able to identify thoughts which produce negative effects on you, and every time you catch a negative
verbal thought as it enters your mind, you can simply remove it by saying "Cancel, cancel". By intercepting negativity while it is still on the mental plane you can prevent
it from being transmuted to the etheric plane, the level of
emotions. By preventing negativity from being transmuted
downward, your feelings will be spared and you will protect
your physical body. If you use this technique conscien-
tiously you can rid yourself of some of the most subtle
forms of negativity.

Once you've stopped negative verbal thoughts from disturbing you, you can go one step further. You can replace fearful thoughts with fearless thoughts; hateful thoughts with loving thoughts, etc. When it comes to thinking in pictures, you can neutralize the effect of negative imagery by replacing it with positive imagery. This should be done without effort and is most easily accomplished when you are in a relaxed mental state.

Let's imagine for a moment this common situation: an employee is called into his boss' office for some unknown reason. His initial reaction is negative, "Did I do something wrong?" he thinks; or even worse, "is my job in jeopardy?" If he continues to entertain these initial thoughts he could trigger a whole avalanche of negative thoughts, which in turn could produce fear and anxiety (remember the worker doesn't know what's going on yet). The initial problem and subsequent problems which could manifest later were caused solely by negative thoughts and imagination. He could neutralize the negative thoughts by saying, "Cancel, cancel". By doing this immediately, he would prevent both a negative emotional response and a negative physical response later. If by chance a negative feeling was already created, the employee could create a positive picture in his mind, and counteract the negative imagery by using positive imagination. By using the techniques described above, the employee could face the situation with a positive attitude rather than a negative one. Furthermore, by using positive imagination he could turn the situation to his advantage. So even if he was called into his boss' office and his first reaction was a negative one, he could turn it around by using "Cancel, cancel". He could affirm, "I am an excellent worker who is appreciated by my superiors", and also, "Every day in every way I'm getting better and better". Finally, he could complete the reprogramming by visualizing himself shaking hands with the boss with both of them smiling at each other.

Positive Affirmations

Below is a list of positive affirmations I have found beneficial in maintaining good health.

1. Every day in every way I'm getting better and better.
2. I can do all things through God, who strengthens me.
3. I have not been given the spirit of fear, but power, love and a sound mind.
4. I am happy; I am healthy; I am whole.
5. I have faith and with faith I can overcome anything.
6. I am complete in every way; filled with courage and inner strength.
7. I am at peace within myself and I accept myself as I am.
8. I am the master of my fate; I am the master of of my life.
9. Negativity has no effect upon me at any level at any time.

You will find that by simply repeating these affirmations to yourself naturally, without effort, they will have a beneficial effect upon you. I suggest you practice one or more of these affirmations ten times a day, out loud if possible, and remind yourself at least once a day that God loves you and with His power nothing can defeat you.

Doubt never accomplishes anything, so if you try reprogramming and at the same time doubt the efficacy of it, you will accomplish very little. If self-doubt is one of your problems, use affirmations and creative imagination to increase your confidence. As most of you know, it doesn't take any effort to think negatively; likewise you needn't exert any effort in order to think positively. I can safely say that the process of reprogramming should be done without effort.

Affirmations "Now"

Thinking occupies so much of a person's time that there are some other aspects of it we should look into. In the physical world there seems to be a sequence of events which humans experience in a lifetime—we call this time. We divide time into past, present and future. This division is based on the reasoning of the conscious mind; and the conscious mind receives the bulk of its information from the five senses. The objective view of time works well while we are conscious, but when we function in the unconscious state, while asleep or in an altered state of mind, the objective view of time breaks down in the same way Newtonian physics breaks down when viewed alongside Einstein's theory of Special Relativity. In the realms of the unconscious there is no past or future; only the present exists. There is no logic or inductive reasoning either. Everything is subjective and is happening "now".

This applies to spiritual healing as well. Healing is always accomplished in the eternal present, in the now. Thus all your affirmations must be asserted in the present tense if they are to have any effect. You should never say, "I will be healed", because this would bring healing into the non existent future; instead, you must say, "Right now I am being healed."

The Electrical Brain

When a person entertains negative thoughts and then as a consequence has a negative emotional and physical response, a change occurs in the brain wave frequency. By understanding the brain and its electrical nature you will get insight into healing on the mental plane.

The human brain generates electricity. There are approximately twenty million brain cells in the human brain, all of which are capable of carrying an electrical charge. Each of these brain cells has an axon which functions as an electrical charge. Each has an axon which functions as an electrical receiver, and between one and twelve transmitters called dentrites. This particular configuration allows for trillions of interconnections between brain cells. When the brain cells are at rest, each cell has a potential electrical force (voltage). When the same cells become active, they release the potential energy and an electric current is generated which carries the message to other nerve cells. The electrical impulses generated by the human brain and the patterns they create have been studied extensively over the past thirty years by an instrument called an electroencephalograph (EEG). EEG patterns can be difficult to understand because brain wave patterns are constantly changing, and no two people have exactly the same patterns.

Although the difference in individual brain wave patterns may be endless, there are general patterns based on brain wave rhythm common to all people and these patterns have been grouped, labeled, and their relationship to different states of consciousness have been uncovered to some extent.

Brain wave rhythms have been grouped into four major categories: *alpha, beta, theta* and *delta*. Alpha was the first brainwave frequency discovered, and it is alpha which is presently causing such a stir. The patterns (rhythms) caused by the brain's electrical activity are measured in cycles per second (CPS). It is generally agreed that about fourteen CPS and higher are known as beta waves, about seven to fourteen are called alpha, four to seven theta, and finally, four and below are delta.

Brainwave patterns cannot be characterized as one specific frequency, because within each category they can vary and that is why they are defined as ranges of frequencies. Different factors can also alter the kind of electrical impulses recorded on an EEG. For example, the placement of the recording electrodes themselves can give different records of brainwave activity depending on whether they are placed on the frontal or pre-central areas of the skull.

A revealing surprise which has come out of biofeedback research is that intense concentrated attention can be present in an individual while his EEG pattern is showing him to be in a state identified as relaxation and inattention.

An individual may exert a great deal of energy in an effort to control his alpha or theta activity, yet his EEG recording will show no sign of unusual effort normally associated with being alert and concentrating on events in the external environment. Could it be possible the EEG is quantitatively showing the qualitative difference between paying attention and concentration, which healers have intuitively discerned for so long?

Delta

The slowest brain wave frequency is called delta. It operates between zero and four cycles per second. Delta appears only during the deepest levels of sleep, in coma or while a person us under anesthesia.

Theta

Theta waves are rarely found in the normal EEG pattern of a human being who is awake. They have a frequency of between four and seven CPS and are associated with drowsiness and the assimilation of new information. Even in the best circumstance, theta waves rarely exceed 5% of the total brain waves discharged during waking hours. They are present most frequently while a person is deeply relaxed or daydreaming. Although theta is normally associated with sleeping, it will suddenly appear during periods of insight or inspiration and during deep healing meditation.

Beta

Once you get above fourteen CPS, above the alpha level, everything is lumped under the heading of beta. Beta activity differs from the others most noticeably because its patterns are often unrhythmic and low voltage. The beta frequency is associated with alert, rational, analytical behavior and concentrated problem solving. It is also accepted that the beta level is a stress state. It is not associated with any particular feeling or state of mind. You could feel anything from fear to joy, happiness to pain

while in beta. However, it has been discovered that negative feelings such as guilt, bitterness, jealousy, fear, etc. are
not found at the lower brain wave frequencies, only at
beta. In addition, research indicates beta is the normal brain
wave pattern of the majority of adults while they are
awake. It is estimated that adults spend 80% of their waking
time in the beta level, while children who have not yet
reached puberty spend 80% of their waking hours in the
alpha state.

Alpha

The alpha level has an electrical frequency of between
seven and fourteen CPS. It is now recognized that increased
alpha production accompanies the practice of both Zen
and Yogic meditation. Students of these disciplines tested
on EEG equipment showed immediate and dramatic increases in quantities of alpha when they began their meditative practice, and after a short while alpha decreased,
only to be replaced by increased theta activity. Many who
reported feeling a sense of separation from the material
universe, loss of personal identity and sense of union
showed the greatest increases in alpha and theta activity.
Being in the alpha level benefits the physical body as well,
because when a person is in the alpha state, the renewing
and self-healing process is accelerated.

Alpha and the Placebo Effect

Increased alpha production has other important features. It increases susceptibility to hypnosis, and hypnosis
makes a person more receptive to suggestion. It follows
that while in the alpha state, a person becomes more receptive to the thoughts, energies and suggestions of people
around him. This phenomenon has important implications
in spiritual healing, since it is now common knowledge that
attitude is an important factor in accelerating the healing
process which is enhanced at the alpha level. For many
years cures which were a product of spiritual healing or
other unorthodox methods were attributed to either

the placebo effect or mind over matter. However, new research shows that the placebo effect and the power of the mind are essential factors in physical healing regardless of what healing procedures are used.

Throughout history, people have been cured by a host of drugs and remedies; everything from crocodile dung to unicorn horn has been used; all of which were worthless in themselves except that the patient expected and believed otherwise and so received benefit from treatment.

As the studies pile up, it becomes clear the placebo effect can be triggered in just about anyone under the right conditions. Albert Schweitzer once said, "The witch doctor succeeds for the same reason all (doctors) succeed . . . each patient carries his own doctor inside him. They come to us not knowing the truth. We are at our best when we give the doctor who resides within each patient a chance to go to work."³⁴

The placebo effect goes beyond pills and injections; it extends even to surgery. A remarkable experiment was conducted in the late '50's and '60's when many surgeons in America began to tie off the mammary arteries of people suffering from angina pectoris, oppressive chest pain, hoping to ease the pains. The results of the operation were extraordinary. Nearly 90% of the patients reported improvement in their condition and concurrent easing of chest pain. But some skeptics doubted the efficacy of the surgery. They believed other factors contributed to the patient's improvement. As a result, an experiment was conducted which today would no longer be considered ethical by American medical standards. Patients were divided into two groups and each patient was told that he would be given an operation which had proven extremely effective in controlling the symptoms of angina pectoris. Half of them actually had the surgery performed, while the other half were given anesthesia, had a small incision made and sutured in their chest; when they were awakened they were told the operation had been a total success. Remarkable as it may seem, when all the results were collected, physicians found that the patients who were given the simulated operation fared better than those who actually underwent surgery.

Alpha and Spiritual Healing
The susceptibility to suggestion which accompanies both the alpha level and which is tied into the placebo effect has some startling implications.

If a human being already has an innate ability to heal himself as scientific research indicates, could it be possible to enhance this ability by entering a particular state of consciousness and by practicing certain healing techniques while at that level? The answer to this question is a resounding yes! When a person is in the alpha/theta level, his own healing ability and ability to heal others is enhanced.

Jose Silva, an early researcher into alpha training, recorded the EEG patterns of psychic and spiritual healers from all over the world and found that while they were engaged in healing, they produced large quantities of alpha waves at ten CPS. More significant was his discovery that patients unconsciously changed their brain wave pattern so it conformed to the brain wave patterns of the healer who worked on them.

We also know that people who function regularly at ten CPS have stronger immunological systems and heal more quickly. They have more control over pain than those who function primarily in the beta level. They can even control involuntary physical responses such as blood pressure, heart rate, body temperature and even bleeding.

By combining affirmations and visualizations while at the alpha level, it is evident people can heal themselves and can also project healing thoughts and energy to others.

The mind can no longer be overlooked. It has clearly emerged today as the principal factor in healing and in maintaining good health.

CHAPTER FIVE

THE ALPHA/THETA STATE

In both the East and West there are traditions of meditation and prayer which effectively stimulate alpha/theta wave production. These practices are usually deeply rooted in tradition and when they are uprooted and taught to us now, they generally serve to confuse rather than enlighten. In spite of these difficulties, simple meditative techniques can be extracted which have no cultural bias and which will be effective in bringing a person into the "alpha/theta state". Once in the alpha/theta state or what is often called the meditative state or light trance state, there is a change in breathing. Breathing tends to become deeper; the heart slows down, the muscles relax and the eyes unfocus. By unfocussing one's eyes, the visual analysis of the external environment is disrupted. The mind is unable to criticize or organize the experiences it receives and shortly stops its attempts to do so. The mind goes blank but not dull, and the emptiness is soon replaced by spontaneous visual images which we call creative imagination or day dreaming. Associated with this state is a strong sense of well-being. Anxiety and worry cease while the mind remains alert and responsive to conscious programming. There is also a growing sensitivity on the left side of the body, especially in the chest cavity, indicating increased activity in the right side of the brain and a more harmonious balance between left hemisphere activity (rational mind) and right hemisphere activity (intuitive mind).

Going into Alpha

To enter the alpha/theta level at will, simply follow these directions. Begin by finding a comfortable position, preferably with your back straight. Take several deep breaths from the abdomen; then close your eyes and relax. Closing the eyes immediately stimulates alpha/theta wave production. Continue breathing deeply and as you do, slowly count backwards from 5 to 1. As you count backwards, mentally repeat and visualize each number three times to yourself. This technique will enhance your ability to visualize, so take your time and let your mind be as creative as it likes. Remember, there is no right way or wrong way to meditate. When you reach number 1, repeat this affirmation to yourself, "I am now deeply relaxed, feeling better than I did before". Continue to breathe deeply and after a few moments begin counting backwards again, this time beginning with the number 10, exhaling as you mentally say 10. Take another deep breath, and while exhaling, mentally repeat the number 9. Take another deep breath, and while exhaling, mentally say 8. Continue in this manner until you have reached number 1. By the time you've reached number 1, you will be feeling very light. Then pay attention to the subtle changes you feel within your body, within your emotions, and of course, within your mind. Each meditation will be different and each time you meditate, you will learn something new about yourself. In meditation you open your energy centers and they in turn permit more energy to enter your "subtle energy system", so unconscious activity is increased.

In many cases physical tension, the tension stored within the muscles, effectively prevents the free flow of energy through the energy centers into the subtle energy system. To release this tension, we use an ancient yogic practice which helps release tension in the voluntary muscles of the body. The Buddhist concept of yin-yang explains that every action has an equal and opposite reaction, so in order to relax and release, you must tighten and contract. After you've reached number 1, mentally repeat this second simple affirmation, "My mind is completely relaxed. Every time I come to this level of mind, I am able to use more of my mind in more creative ways". Then, rest in this state for a few moments. When you feel ready, bring your attention to your feet; draw in your breath and contract the muscles of your feet as much as possible. Hold your breath for three seconds. After three seconds, release your breath and allow the muscles of your feet to relax. Inhale deeply again and repeat the procedure, this time with your ankles and calves. Continue by repeating the same procedure with the following parts of your body : the thighs, the buttocks and pelvis, the middle and upper abdomen, the chest and shoulders, the neck, the arms, and then the hands. Then squeeze the muscles of your face and hold for three seconds. After three seconds, release and exhale. Next, open your mouth, stick out your tongue and stretch the muscles of your face as much as possible; hold your breath for three seconds, then release the muscles of your face and exhale.

To complete the exercise, contract your entire body (this time squeezing the muscles of your face), and hold your breath. Finally, after three seconds, expel the air forcibly through your nose while releasing all the muscles of your body at once.

Ten to fifteen minutes will have elapsed by this time, and you should be firmly in the "alpha/theta level". Then mentally affirm, "I am in the alpha level. Every time I come to this level of mind, it makes it easier for me to go to deeper and healthier levels."

Pay attention to your physical body and feel the subtle vibrations and energies which flow through it. Continue paying attention for a few moments more and observe the spontaneous images flowing through your mind. Make no attempt to control them; simply observe them, watch them, but don't get attached to them. As you flow with these images, allow your mind to drift to its sanctuary, its perfect place of relaxation. Your sanctuary is a place with no appointments to keep, no bills to pay, no stress to disturb you. It is a place where you feel content and free from anxiety, doubts, insecurities, etc. and where you are at peace with yourself and the environment around you. It doesn't matter whether it is somewhere on earth or a place that you create on the mental plane. The important thing is that it becomes a place of sanctuary (a place for renewal) for you during times of stress. So, while you're there, enjoy yourself and relax completely. I suggest you remain in your sanctuary for about five minutes. Keep your senses and emotions awake and open, and experience your sanctuary as completely as you can.

So far I have illustrated a simple and effective technique for relaxation, for bringing your mind into the alpha/theta level. However, once you are in the alpha/theta level, you can direct your attention towards reprogramming yourself and later for healing. We perfect our ability to visualize and heal mentally through a technique called mental projection. While at the alpha/theta level, you can project your consciousness anywhere in the universe you want to through affirmations and visualizations. Not only can you go anywhere you want, but you can use mental projection to heal yourself in any facet of your life.

The Mental Projection

Once you have returned from your sanctuary, you can begin projecting your consciousness by mentally affirming, "I can project my consciousness anywhere in the universe I want". Then take a deep breath while continuing to breathe deeply through your nose without separation between inhalation and exhalation. Next, put your palms together over your heart, in the same way that saints in the early church are depicted (see plate) and continue breathing deeply while you bring your attention to your third eye. It is the center of higher intelligance from which we receive and project visual images. It is located just above the bridge of the nose and between the eyebrows. None of these tasks require any effort. Simply breathe deeply and rhythmically, and put your palms together over your heart.

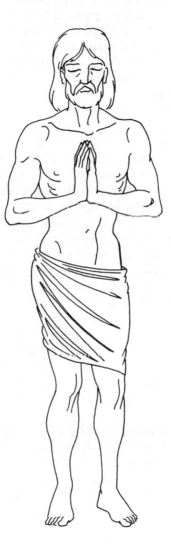

Plate 2: The Saint Position

This will stimulate your heart and will help you in visualization. It also neutralizes the physical body's magnetic charge, which can disrupt your ability to visualize. Once your attention is on the third eye, you are ready to begin visualization and mental projection. You can perfect your ability to project your consciousness and to visualize by projecting your consciousness into the three levels of matter on the physical plane; the mineral kingdom, the vegetable kingdom, and the animal kingdom.

Before you begin mental projection, remember that once you have prepared the centers of consciousness within you by entering the alpha/theta level, you must accept the possibility of mental projection. This shouldn't be difficult because you are continually performing mental projection while dreaming at night and during the day when you are daydreaming or using your imagination. When you are imagining yourself in a particular place or situation, you are actually going to it as it exists on the mental plane. Everything that exists on the physical plane—as we know from the first Hermetic axiom—had a prior existence on the mental plane before it was transmuted to the physical plane. So, don't be confused; mental projection is not merely imagination. When you see spontaneous images while at the alpha/theta level, you see things that are real and that exist on the mental plane; and when you reprogram by creating new images, you are creating new realities on the mental plane which later will be transmuted into physical reality.

Let's begin our exercise by projecting our consciousness into the simplest form of matter in the physical world; inanimate matter found in the mineral kingdom. Then, we will move on to the kingdoms of greater complexity.

Continue to breathe deeply and then visualize a platform about three feet high and located between six and nine feet in front of you. On that platform visualize a large brown rock about three feet in diameter. Keep your senses open and active as you observe the rock, because using the five senses is just as important on the mental plane as it is on the physical plane. (Some people mistakenly believe there is a sixth sense which is used exclusively to experience the higher planes. This is not exactly the case. The sixth sense is no more than human intuition, which the healer calls clairsentience. He uses clairsentience along with his five senses to gather information from the higher planes.)

After you have examined the stone from six feet away and have observed its size, shape, color and texture, visualize yourself standing beside it close enough to reach out and touch it. Then visualize yourself touching it. This will allow you to use more than your sight alone. You will be able to see the stone in greater detail now; you will be able to touch the stone, to feel its texture, temperature as well as its smoothness and dampness, etc. Details are very important in mental projection and in healing, and the more qualities of an object you can experience the better. Therefore, take a minute or two to examine the stone from close up; take a deep breath and mentally affirm, "I am now inside the stone and I am experiencing it in its fullness." In that instant, you will find yourself inside the stone, in an appropriate size to fit comfortably. While you are inside, take your time and explore the stone. You can change your size by just willing it, so it is possible for you to explore the inside of the rock even on the molecular level. While inside the stone, you will be able to use all of your senses psychically. You will be able to see, hear, taste, smell, and touch; experiencing the qualities of the stone completely.

Besides using your senses, use your intuition to feel the spirit of the stone; what can be called the essence of it. All things created have this individual "essential" quality and by experiencing this quality, a healer can actually sense the rightness or wrongness of its vibration. Feeling in this way is extremely important in healing, because in the psychic diagnosis of disease, a sense of wrongness is often the first indication of a negative vibration and disease in a person's "subtle energy system".

I suggest that in the beginning you take three or four minutes to explore the inside of the stone. After a short time or when you are satisfied you have experienced the stone in its fullness, visualize yourself standing outside of it again, about six feet in front of the platform. Then mentally release the stone. Take a deep breath while keeping your palms together and go deeper (relax more completely).

We will mentally project into the plant kingdom next. Keep your palms together and with your attention on your third eye, visualize a pot of tulips on the platform in front of you. Each time you visualize something from the physical world, repeat the process you learned from examining the stone. Of course, as you progress you can substitute different objects from each of the kingdoms. But for now, simply observe the tulips from six feet away. Take a few moments for this and then visualize yourself standing next to the flowers. Reach out with your hand as you did before and touch them. Remember to keep your senses and feelings awake and active when you experience the plant. Take a few moments to examine the tulips close up. Then, take a deep breath and mentally repeat the affirmation, "I am inside the tulips, experiencing them in their fullness." You will instantaneously find yourself inside the plant. I suggest you begin your exploration of the tulip with the flower, examining the organs of the flower, then moving down to the stem and finally completing the examination with the roots. Since you are dealing with a more complex living thing, take your time and experience not only the physical qualities of the plant, but try to get in touch with the "life force" which flows through it. The life force is a manifestation of prana, the "absolute energy". I suggest you take about five minutes or more to complete your examination of the plant. When you have experienced it in its fullness, visualize yourself outside the plant again about six feet in front of the platform. Then, release the plant, take a deep breath and feel yourself relaxing even more (going deeper). If you prefer you can practice each of these mental projections as a separate meditation and exercise, or as we are doing here, you can substitute one object or living thing for another while remaining in the alpha/theta level; experiencing them in sequence. If you are not tired and can maintain your attention for an extended period of time, continue with the sequence as I present it here, because later when you learn the techniques of absentee healing, you may want to heal more than one person during a healing meditation and this would require substituting one person for another in the same way we are projecting consciousness now. If you want to end the meditation after one or two mental projections, follow the instructions at the end of this chapter.

From mental projection in the vegetable kingdom, we proceed to mental projection in the animal kingdom. By moving up on the evolutionary scale, we can make "contact" with your subject on more levels. In the animal kingdom, not only can you experience the physical qualities and the "life force" of the creature you are examining, but you can experience its emotions and animal consciousness as well.

To continue this meditation breathe deeply while keeping your hands together above your heart. When you are ready, visualize an animal on the platform. A household pet is your best bet; however, you can visualize any animal you are familiar with, either a farm animal or an animal you've seen at a zoo or in the wild. Visualize the animal on the platform and examine its physical body from top to bottom. After a few moments visualize yourself standing next to the animal and then reach out and begin stroking it. Be attentive to the creature's reaction. You can learn much about your subject in this way. Continue using all of your senses, but even more than before begin feeling the distinct personality of the animal you are making contact with. It is important to remember that you are using more than your imagination when you project your consciousness. You are making contact with the animal on the mental level through your unconscious mind. The animal in

question will feel your presence so be gentle. It may help
to speak mentally with the creature to reassure it of your
positive intentions. Empathy is an important part of healing, so begin here to empathize with the animal you are
making contact with. You will find this easy to do if you
begin role playing, allowing yourself to sense the feelings
of the creature, and if possible to think its thoughts. When
you feel satisfied that you have experienced both the physical qualities and the personality of the animal, take a deep
breath and mentally affirm, "I am now inside the animal,
experiencing it in its fullness." Instantaneously you will find
yourself inside the animal in the appropriate size to fit
comfortably. I suggest you begin your examination of the
animal with the lungs. Visualize yourself standing between
them and using all your senses, begin your examination.
Reach out your hand and touch one of them. You will feel
the rhythmic movement of the lungs as the animal breathes
in and out. Experience all the physical qualities you can
but don't stop there; feel the rightness or wrongness of the
lungs, ask yourself the question: are the lungs functioning
normally, are they healthy and in harmony? Lastly, empathize with the creature and through role reversal experience
yourself as the animal. The ability to experience something
completely is an acquired skill; so is the ability to empathize. Do the best you can and don't be discouraged if you
can't experience the animal in its fullness right away. With
practice, you will. When you have experienced the lungs
and the area around them to your satisfaction, project
yourself to the base of the animal's spinal column. Reach
out and touch one of the vertebra. Notice the difference
between the different tissue and organs in the spinal area.
Take two to three minutes to examine the vertebra, spinal
column and surrounding tissue. After two or three minutes
or when you feel satisfied, project yourself to any place
you like within the animal's body. If you go to a diseased
area, notice the differences between healthy and diseased
tissue. Then, take another four or five minutes to complete
your examination. When you are finished, visualize yourself

outside the animal, six feet in front of the platform. Take a deep breath and mentally release the animal and the platform. Put your hands down at your sides and relax.

In succeeding meditations, you can continue examining the same animal or a different animal if you like. I suggest you practice mental projection regularly from now on, since many of our techniques in spiritual healing are dependent on it.

Your return trip to normal consciousness begins with an affirmation. While breathing deeply and rhythmically, mentally affirm, "Every time I go to this level of mind, it makes it easier for me to go to deeper and healthier levels of mind." Then slowly begin counting from 1 to 5 this way: 1, 2, then mentally say, "I am coming up slowly" . . . . count 3, 4, 5, . . . open your eyes . . . and when you reach 5, say to yourself, "I feel wide awake, perfectly relaxed and better than I did before."

CHAPTER SIX

THE CHAKRAS

The energy from the spiritual, mental and etheric planes which we use for healing enters the physical plane through energy centers called *chakras*.

The energy from the higher planes directly affects our emotions and our physical health. Each of us has seven chakras (the word chakra in Sanskrit means wheel). They appear within us as wheel-like openings on the surface of our etheric body. In actuality, they look like long, thin funnels with the larger opening on the surface of the etheric body. They resemble the old hearing devices used in the nineteenth century. (See plate 1)

These chakras act as terminals through which energy (prana) is transferred from the higher planes to the physical body. An understanding of the way they function is essential for the understanding and practice of spiritual healing. In the same way that problems occur in modern rail and air terminals when traffic becomes clogged, problems may occur when energy becomes clogged as it is transferred through the chakras. These problems, which originate on the higher planes, weaken the subtle energy system. The weakness is then transmuted to the physical plane and it creates fertile ground for the development of physical disease.

The clairvoyant will often see or feel disease in the etheric plane before it becomes manifest in the physical body. He can see it clairvoyantly using his psychic ability, he can feel it with his hand, or he can see it in his patient's aura (the energy field surrounding and permeating each human being). In October 1982, a young woman came to me for a psychic consultation, and in the course of it I clairvoyantly saw a large man who appeared to be in his fifties, balding and who wore glasses. He seemed to be related to her. I asked her about him and she replied that her father-in-law fit the description. I asked her about his heart condition since I could see a brown patch in the aura above his heart. Brown in the aura always indicates disease. She replied that he had no heart problem and in his last checkup two months earlier, the doctors declared that he was in perfect health. I explained to her that the disease although not yet manifested in the physical body certainly existed and would sooner or later affect him negatively. She remained unconvinced and left shortly afterwards. Six weeks later, I received a phone call; it was the same young woman. She called to ask if I would perform an absentee healing for her father-in-law who had just suffered a heart attack. She explained that he was in the hospital under intensive care and that she would be greatly encouraged if I worked on him which of course I did. Fortunately he recovered, but was forced to restrict his activities from that time on.

This man's heart attack might have been prevented if at the time I saw his condition, I had been permitted to work with him and teach him how to open and balance his chakras. (Good health is not possible unless chakras are functioning properly.) Perhaps then his heart disease would not have been transmuted from the etheric plane to the physical plane.

In order to rectify problems in the chakras and prevent the development of disease, I have developed a simple exercise which when used regularly will open and balance the chakras so energy will flow smoothly through them. The process of opening and balancing the chakras has a dual purpose. First, it is necessary to keep your chakras open and balanced to maintain your own good health. If a person does have medical problems, bringing the chakras into balance will promote his rapid healing and recovery. Second, healing others requires the transfer of large amounts of energy through the chakras. This can only be done when they are open and well balanced.

In my workshops, I have discovered that by preparing students properly beforehand by having them open and balance their chakras before they begin channeling healing energy to their patients, they can achieve far greater success than if they begin healing with their chakras shut down and unbalanced. I have found that in my practice when I pray and meditate regularly, practices which keep the chakras healthy and strong, I have far greater success in healing.

The First Chakra

As I said before, there are seven chakras. The first, or root chakra is located at the base of the spine and is fiery orange-red when active. It is a channel for subtle energies entering the earth plane, and when it is functioning properly a person feels a deep personal attachment to the earth. The seven chakras are associated with the seven major glands within the physical body. Alice Bailey states, "The seven centers of force are to be found in the same region where the seven major glands are located and each center of force, according to the esoteric teaching . . . is in fact, its externalization."[35] The first chakra corresponds to the adrenal glands. As we know, the adrenal glands control the chemical constitution of body fluids; they lie one above each kidney.

The Second Chakra

The second chakra is alternately known as the sacral or splenic chakra. It is situated in the neighborhood of the reproductive organs. This chakra corresponds to the sun and therefore when active radiates all the colors of the vital force (prana): red, orange, yellow, blue and violet. It is associated with the gonads and controls both sexual and creative energy.

The Third Chakra

The third chakra is alternately known as the naval or solar plexus center. Its importance lies in the fact that through it we feel connected to the physical and etheric world. It is the outlet through which our emotional energy flows. For the average person, it is the seat of the personality. It is associated with two colors, red and green. The solar plexus chakra corresponds to the pancreas, a flat organ which lies behind and slightly below the stomach. The enzymes secreted from the pancreas are important in the metabolism of fats and proteins. Furthermore, the pancreas secretes insulin, which is of profound importance in balancing blood sugar levels and controlling carbohydrate metabolism.

The Fourth Chakra

The fourth chakra is the heart center; it is a glowing, golden color. It is the source of light and love, not only of human love, but agape love, the Divine love which the New Testament so poetically describes as "rivers of living water."[36] The heart chakra is of utmost importance in healing. It is from the human heart that " . . . the love of God is shed abroad."[37] The transforming energies of the heart are a major focal point in the study of healing. We must learn to think from the heart, projecting our consciousness from that vital center, thereby focusing powerful healing rays to those who need healing. The heart chakra is located just over the heart. The thymus gland corresponds with the heart chakra; so far, not much is known about its workings, however, modern research connects it with the immunological system, and although it attains its greatest size during puberty and then the lymphatic tissue is replaced by simple fatty tissue, there is reason to believe its stimulation enhances and stimulates the immunological system well into adulthood.

The Fifth Chakra

The fifth chakra is known as the throat chakra. To the

trained clairvoyant it appears silvery blue, oftentimes with a hint of green. The center is found in the back of the neck, starting just below the medulla oblongata and reaching downwards toward the front of the throat just below the Adam's apple. This chakra is important because it is the center of human expression; permitting each entity to communicate creatively with the outside world. It transmits the intent of the soul. Its physical externalization is the thyroid gland, which guards body equilibrium by controlling the rate of metabolism. It is found on both sides of the trachea.

The Sixth Chakra

The sixth chakra is alternately called the brow chakra, or the Third Eye. It is located directly between and slightly above the eyebrows. It radiates with two primary colors; yellow, alternating with a deep blue which in the developed personality borders on violet. It is directly related to seeing; not only in the physical sense, but in the mystical sense of seeing into the higher planes; intuitive seeing, clairvoyance and the other paranormal forms of knowing. It is the seat of creativity and when active and open, the seat of Divine intelligence. It is of paramount importance in absentee healing.

In my work, I have found that channeling rays from both the brow chakra (the Third Eye) and the heart chakra simultaneously is an effective way to transmit healing from a distance. In my workshops, I explain that when I activate these two chakras mentally and physically, and then visualize the rays from them being absorbed by my patient, the rays have a pronounced effect on them.

The brow chakra's physical externalization is the pituitary gland, which is located at the base of the skull and which secretes several hormones whose general overall function is to regulate growth and metabolism.

The Seventh Chakra

The seventh chakra is known as the crown chakra.

When active, it is the most vibrant of them all. It seems to vibrate with a host of colors, yet to the trained eye it is predominantly violet. It is located at the very top of the head and is called the "thousand petalled lotus" in Hindu scripture. It is the last chakra to be awakened and therefore corresponds to the highest level of spiritual perfection. Like the other chakras, it is a channel for higher energies, which enter each of us from the higher planes; however, unlike the others, when fully active it can reverse itself, and then it radiates like a central sun, showering love and largess into the surrounding environment. The crown chakra corresponds to the pineal gland, which is located on the underside of the midbrain. Its function is not fully understood in medical terms, but there is evidence it is concerned with growth; beyond that, little is known. Its importance for us lies in the fact that it is the recipient of the most profound spiritual energies and it is precisely these energies which have a transforming affect on physical disease. The energies which enter through the crown are renewable; and as more spiritual force is generated for the work of regeneration, more energy flows into the chakra, forming above the head of the individual a veritable crown of pure light and Divine energy.

A short time after I gave myself totally to my healing practice, I began to notice that during and after a healing session, my head would glow or vibrate with the center of the vibration coming from the top of my head radiating downward through my skull. The more I worked, the more pronounced the glow became until it seemed to last all day—then for days on end—growing stronger whenever I paid attention to it. It was an extremely pleasant feeling, but it puzzled me until I was reminded by some associates about the particular properties of the crown chakra, (that the energies can reverse themselves) and many healers have experienced this glowing sensation and that once the reaction had begun, usually through performing some sort of spiritual service, the energy became self-generating.

Opening and Balancing the Chakras

The chakras, as we have seen, are openings which transmit energy to our physical body; each chakra is a doorway for energy of a different frequency. When any of these doorways is closed or blocked for any reason whatsoever, problems arise because energy needed to nourish the physical body is restricted, and these problems will later be transmuted into physical disease. In order to correct these problems, you must open and balance the seven chakras. The technique I've described below, when practiced regularly, will do just that. I call it "chakra balancing".

Begin by finding a quiet place where you can sit or lie comfortably for about five minutes. It makes no difference if you sit or lie down. Just make sure your back is straight. For those of you familiar with the lotus position, it will suffice; if you have trouble with it, finding it uncomfortable for any reason, your results will be equally good if you lie on your back with your hands at your sides. So, find a comfortable position either sitting in the lotus position, sitting in a straight backed chair, or lying on your back. Then simply close your eyes and relax. Let your mind wander and make no effort to control it, but instead let it go to its perfect place of relaxation (your sanctuary).

Let yourself rest there for awhile, and then count backward from 5 to 1, and on each descending number take a long deep breath and feel yourself drifting deeper. There is no need to control the mind in any way, but simply let it go where it likes.When you've reached the number 1, silently repeat the affirmation, "I am deeply relaxed, feeling better than I did before." As you can see, during every spiritual exercise we take the opportunity to reprogram ourselves. Then pay attention to the first chakra, which is at the base of your spine. As soon as you pay attention to it, the chakra will begin to vibrate and tingle. That's how you can locate each chakra; the tingling sensation originates from its center. By paying attention to your chakras you will experience them opening and expanding. You can feel the very spot where they are located and the pulsating, tingling sensation caused by the energies passing through them into your aura.

By paying attention to the first chakra, not only can you locate it, but the mental force of your attention serves to activate it. This mental stimulation is the first step in opening the chakras. The next step is breathing from each individual chakra. In this way you can stimulate them even further by bringing the energy inherent in the breath, which is a manifestation of "prana" (the vital force) to the chakras. With these two tools, the mind and the breath, at your service, you can easily initiate the process of opening and balancing your energy centers. Begin at the first chakra (base of the spine) by mentally paying attention to it. Next, breathe into it, and then without separation between inhalation and exhalation, breathe out, and as you do chant the universal OHM from the chakra.* The important thing to remember in the last stage (chanting on the exhalation) is that the musical note you chant must cause a sympathetic vibration in the chakra. We can liken this phenomenon to the sympathetic vibration which results in a violin when a tuning fork is struck which has the same tone as one of the strings. Repeat the process of chanting OHM three times from each chakra, starting at the base of the spine and ending at the crown.

Raise the OHM one note for each chakra, beginning with G for the first chakra, going through the seven notes of the scale (as you go through the seven chakras). The technique of chakra balancing takes only three to four minutes, but even in such a short time the results can be remarkable. Not only are the chakras opened, but they are balanced, creating a healthy integration of energies which in turn strengthen and revitalize the physical body's energy system. The subtle energy system is strengthened

---

*OHM in Sanskrit is the sound of the universal vibration. This is the sound uttered by God at the creation and which is the combined sound of all created things.

also, which safeguards you from negativity encountered from both your internal and external environment. Many people compare its effects to the effects of meditating for a half hour or more. I often recommend it as an alternative when time is unavailable for a more lengthy meditation. It should ideally be practiced twice a day, in the morning and late afternoon. I don't recommend practicing it around bedtime, since it tends to stimulate the nerves and can keep you awake. If you practice it regularly you will soon begin to experience its effects. Your mind will become more alert and you will experience less idle chatter and static running through it. Anxiety will decrease and you will feel more relaxed. Furthermore, your energy level will increase, filling you with a greater sense of well-being. The practice stimulates the flow of prana into your physical body, allowing your body to heal and renew itself more quickly. You will be more useful and more successful as a channel for healing since more prana will be flowing through you. As always, by healing yourself, you will become more effective in healing others.

CHAPTER SEVEN

PRANA

Prana in Sanskrit means "absolute energy" (the vital force). It is believed that with each breath a person takes, in flows prana. By becoming a Master of Pranayama, the Science of Breath, a person can learn not only to control his breath, but he can immerse himself in the vital force and can then learn to control his "subtle energy system", so he can transmute energy into any vibration he requires. This vital force acts like a cosmic glue. It radiates from the All, flowing into each dimension, filling all available space, connecting everything on all four levels. It is the primordial force which is the source of all forces in the Universe; it is the primordial energy which is at the source of all energy in the Universe; it transmits thought through the ether and yet—it is not thought! It is not matter, but because of it (prana) matter exists, with all its variations. Everything that "is" springs from prana as it is transmuted into different vibrations. Yet, prana is not consciousness (Brahma), prana is simply the absolute energy which keeps everything going, which is the fuel of life.

In the *Bhagavad Gita*, we are told that the yogi can become a master of Pranayama and by so doing he can become one with Brahma . . . becoming a co-creator in the All's continuing creation. Using the vital force along with his unconscious mind he can renew what is neglected and heal what is diseased. His mastery enables him to transmute anything he wants " . . . from state to state; degree to

67

degree; condition to condition . . ."[38]
Prana is likened to fire in the *Kathopanisad*:

> Listen, O Naciteka, listen with all attention.
> I have the knowledge of fire
> which leads the way to immortality.
> It is indeed the path to heaven,
> this fire—this energy.
> It is the support of all creation,
> and it is rooted deep within the cave of heart
> (the mystery of life).[39]

When a person becomes a master of pranayama, he can use the "absolute energy" to renew, to create, and most importantly, to heal. It is the breath which carries prana in its most concentrated form through a person's "subtle energy system", and it is through proper breathing that you can increase your energy level (level of prana) and then use the prana like you would electricity for any useful purpose.

Natural Breathing

The breath is responsible for more than just bringing oxygen into the body. It largely determines a person's state of health by determining the quantity and quality of prana which flows into the subtle energy system from the higher realms. By paying attention (by seeing himself clearly) the healer learns the importance of proper breathing. He sees that improper breathing disrupts the normal flow of energy and nourishment coming from the higher planes into his physical body. Divine energy (prana) may be transmuted into lower vibrations, but it originates on the spiritual plane, and for our purposes is synonymous with the Divine healing force which comes from God, the All.

Improper breathing inhibits the healing process, and when I speak of the healing process, I mean the self-healing or renewing process as well. To maintain proper health, a person must breathe properly. When the breath is not complete; when it is shallow, when a person breathes through the mouth, when a person unconsciously holds the breath between inhalation and exhalation, that person disrupts his system on the physical level; but more importantly, he disrupts the free flow of prana traveling through the chakras. On the physical level, shallow breathing weakens the muscles of the diaphragm through disuse. Improper breathing also weakens the lower third of the lungs for the same reason. Improper breathing inhibits the free flow of energy from the etheric level and consequently the emotions are suppressed. Shallow breathing also disrupts the emotions of love and belonging which are associated with the third and fourth chakras; the solar plexus and the heart respectively. Because prana cannot reach the third and fourth chakras, a person's relationships and his connection with the world, his connection to institutions, people and places is disrupted.

In the case of the fourth chakra, the heart center, it is love which is inhibited. The danger should be obvious. When you habitually take shallow breaths, you cut off love, warmth and tenderness; as a result you feel isolated in a world where real fulfillment comes almost exclusively from loving relationships. Moreover, any disease on the etheric level, the level of emotions, will be eventually transmuted, resulting in disease on the physical level.

Those of you who spend time around small children may have noticed that children breathe without separation between inhalation and exhalation; this is natural, proper breathing. Children don't learn to breathe this way, it is a natural rhythm which functions beautifully until something comes along to disrupt it. The healer, through his work, becomes "childlike" — he remembers his natural rhythms and allows his body to return to them. For those of you who notice a slight pause between inhalation and exhalation, practice the exercise at the end of this chapter. It will help you to re-educate your body and you will remember to breathe like a child in the healthiest way possible. That little separation might seem insignificant, but it can have a disruptive effect on the fifth chakra (the throat chakra) as well. It inhibits self-expression which often causes anxiety and self-consciousness.

Breathing from the mouth is another abnormal form of respiration. It can be injurious for several reasons. By neglecting to use the normal breathing organs, a person bypasses the filters amd dust catchers within the body. Instead of having dust, impurities and foreign objects trapped by the mucous membranes and the hairs of the nostrils, mouth breathing gives foreign particles direct access to the entire respiratory system. These particles can become lodged in the respiratory system and they can accumulate there, irritating the bronchial tubes and lungs. This irritation can cause inflammation and even greater problems later on. The nasal passages have another important function, cooling hot air and warming cold air as it enters the body. When you breathe from the mouth, air can enter your respiratory system at extreme termperatures and this can damage the system. Yogi Ramacharaka says that a person who habitually breathes through the mouth is " . . .violating one of nature's laws and is sowing the seeds of disease."[40]

By going through the long narrow nasal passages as it ought to, air is not only cleansed of particles and brought to the correct temperature, it is purified and immediately begins releasing prana into the system. Mouth breathing has another negative feature; by breathing through the mouth, you neglect the nasal passages and through disuse, they become clogged and unclean. This unhealthy condition can lead to local problems such as congestion, inflammation and infection.

Yogic Breathing

In Yoga, there is a technique which will help you "remember" to breathe properly. This technique is called the three part Yogic breath. I will break it down for you in a moment, but first let me say that I am really asking you to remember something you already know. I'm not teaching you anything new. If we put things in their proper perspective, you would see that people learn how to be ill. For most of us our original state was one of perfect harmony and health. Being sick is a process which continues only so long as a person lends it his conscious and unconscious support.

Being sick is not a static state of being. It is a process; it is fluid, continuing only as long as you nourish it. By removing your support, you can reverse the process. Once you stop feeding it, once you alter the conditions necessary to keep it going, it (the disease) will starve and eventually disappear.

When you breathe properly, you bring nourishment and vitality into your system. The vital force (prana) helps the body mobilize its resources against disease. With greater force mobilized against it, the disease is forced to respond to less harmonious conditions within the body.

The full breath, what I call the Yogic Breath, is a synthesis of the three basic breaths and is often called the complete breath. The three elements are: the abdominal breath in which the abdomen is expanded and stretched downward; the mid-breath in which air, once having filled the abdomen, expands to fill the chest cavity, expanding the rib cage and lifting the shoulders; and the nasal breath, in which air, having first filled the abdomen and then the chest, fills the nasal passages and continues filling the head. In complete Yogic breathing, not only do you bring more oxygen into your physical body, but you stimulate the chakras by bringing prana down through the abdomen and up to the top of the head. As you know, everything vibrates, including prana, and its vibration affects the chakras, helping to keep them open and functioning harmoniously.

Correct breathing is an essential part of the other techniques mentioned in this book. So, I encourage every one of you to take time each day and practice the exercise described below. You will find it very beneficial.

Begin by sitting in a comfortable position with your back straight and your legs flat on the floor. You can use the lotus position if you like. Once you're sitting comfortably, place your right hand on your abdomen just below the solar plexus. This will help you feel the rhythm of your breath and will make it more fluid and rhythmic. Then close your eyes. Closing the eyes is not essential, but it will help you to relax, making rhythmic breathing easier. Begin by breathing in; first filling your lower lungs with air. With your hand on your abdomen, you will feel the muscles of your diaphragm stretch as your stomach becomes slightly extended. Continue breathing inward, feeling the air fill the middle and upper part of your lungs. Your shoulders will lift and the muscles of the rib cage will stretch as the lungs expand. During the mid-breath, some people feel pain in the upper back between the shoulder blades. The pain is caused by muscles which over the years have contracted and have become stiff. This is largely due to improper breathing. Don't let a little discomfort discourage you, press on; in a few days the discomfort will disappear and your muscles will return to their normal state of elasticity. After air has filled your lungs, let it continue to rise, filling your nasal passages and head, giving you a light pleasant sensation. When you exhale, reverse the process, letting the nasal passages empty first and then the upper, mid, and finally the lower lungs. Your shoulders will naturally drop and the diaphragm will then return to its normal position. (See plate) Without separation between inhalation and exhalation, continue this exercise for about five minutes. At first, reserve special times during the day for practice, but once the rhythm is mastered, you should make this form of breathing the norm. Become attentive to your breathing and gently bring it back to the complete breath every time it becomes shallow or falls into an old habit. Now, A NOTE OF WARNING: be sure that you are gentle with yourself! Don't fall victim to watching yourself and your breathing all the time. Don't become obsessive about it, becuase you will simply undermine yourself in other areas, and instead of liberating yourself, you will restrict yourself even more.

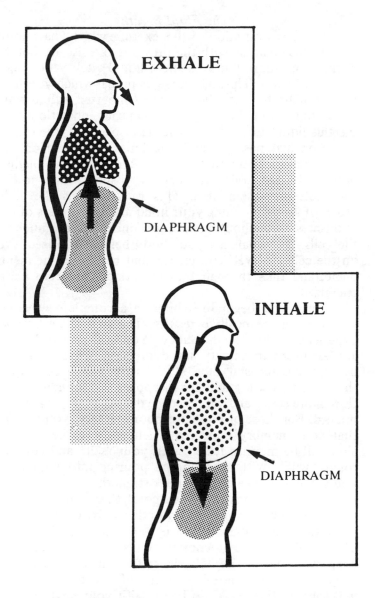

Plate 3: The Yogic Breath

The Fluid Breath

There is a variation of this exercise which I have found useful. It is identical with the previous exercise, except that during inhalation, you imagine a liquid vitality flowing in with the breath. This, of course, is prana, which you see in your visualization as a liquid, or even better, a fluid which is bursting with light and energy. On each inhalation, imagine this liquid flowing into the nasal passages, the sinuses, the bronchial passages and the lungs, and then on each exhalation, imagine that energy is radiating throughout your body, recharging the organs, tissues, cells, and even the molecules themselves. This variation has the added effect of reprogramming your mind and the centers of consciousness throughout your body, including the nuclei of the cells. By visualizing your body being revitalized, even on the cellular level, you create that reality on the mental plane, and then through transmutation, your cells are re-energized.

Once you begin breathing in a complete way, you should soon see positive results. The first thing you will experience is increased vitality. You will notice that you are less prone to anxiety and depression. What's more, the nervous chatter and morbid thoughts which accompany those feelings will gradually disappear. Your emotions will flow more easily and will become deeper as the chakras are opened. For those of you with poor memory, you will find that your memory improves when you breathe properly. You will be more in touch with your "self" and your personal "will". With more prana pouring into your body, you will experience greater inner strength and more energy. With increased prana at your disposal, there is more strength to overcome bad habits and addictive activities will quickly fall away. The Yogic breath is especially useful for those of you who are heavy smokers. Once you begin breathing properly, your desire for cigarettes will drop markedly. Proper breathing underlies many of the techniques you will learn in this book. So begin with your next breath to breathe deeply and completely, and from then on, acquire the habit of breathing properly. If you do, you will never again go back to your bad breathing habits.

CHAPTER EIGHT

ABSENTEE HEALING

As you progress in healing you will become more aware of your inner environment. You will learn more about the I AM, your unconscious "self". You will experience more prana flowing through your "subtle energy system", the system which channels and distributes energy; you will find it easier to pay attention and then you will begin to remember who you are. The re-awakening and liberation of your unconscious "self" is essential for success in healing. When you have come back into balance by refusing to identify exclusively with your lower (conscious) self, then you can become an agent of Divine consciousness, and can act as a channel for healing energy. Then, your charisma, the mark of your new balance, will become evident to everyone you meet, and wherever you go, you will bring healing. "If one really wishes to be master of an art . . . (in our case healing) . . . technical knowledge is not enough." The contemporary Zen master D. T. Suzuki tells us, "One has to transcend technique so that art becomes an artless art growing out of the unconsciousness."[41]

You already know from earlier chapters that the mind thinks in words while at the beta frequency, the conscious level. You also know that it thinks in pictures when the brain wave frequency slows down to the alpha/theta level. It is while you are at the alpha/theta level, the unconscious level, that you are continually being healed and renewed; also, it is from this level that healing energy flows most readily between one person and another.

Focusing Healing Energy

As you know, human beings, through mental visualization, can project their consciousness anywhere in the universe they want. Also, through mental projection they can alter physical reality by creating new realities on the mental plane through visualization. Moreover, the ability to visualize allows a person to focus mental (healing) energies to those who require healing. You can liken visualization to daydreaming except that in visualization, unlike daydreaming, images are not generated at random but are programmed consciously through affirmations prior to or during a healing session. The conscious mind, i. e. the rational objective mind, can be thought of as a computer keyboard. Through it a person can program in, or in other words affirm what he wants and from the central date bank, what Edgar Cayce called the Akashic Records and what Carl Jung called the Collective Unconscious Mind, information in the form of images will appear on the screen of the conscious mind. We can take this natural ability to program images and we can develop from it a technique that can universally be applied in healing. With it you will learn to direct healing energies to those who need them.

Experiencing Alpha

You already have a reliable method for entering the alpha/theta level at will. This is important in healing because healing is more than affirmations and visualization. Healing is the channeling of spiritual energy (which comes from the All) by the healer (while he is at the alpha/theta level). It will not belabor the point to remind you again that those who channel energy from the All, the source of healing are not the healers; they simply channel and focus the energy which comes through them.

But to focus this energy there must be a rapport between the source of healing, the All, and the channel, who we call for convenience, the healer. The process of focusing healing energy through the mind or from the mental plane for use in physical healing is the subject of this chapter. In this chapter we will combine the breathing and meditation techniques which you already know with mental projection to create a technique called the "visual screen". You can use the visual screen for healing as long as you are in rapport with the All, the source of healing energy.

Surrender

Healing grows out of the unconscious when a person is in rapport with the healing source. It is the ego, a function of the conscious mind, which blocks the experience of this rapport. The healer must unseat the ego without crushing it in order to open the doors to healing energy. Only then can rapport be established. Achieving rapport is accomplished by an act of surrender on the part of the healer; when the healer pushes aside the ago to make room for the I AM.

Surrender is a process which always happens in the "now" but must be repeated many times for it to be impressed deeply within a person. It can be accelerated through meditation, yogic breathing, visualization and particularly through affirmations. The more you affirm that you want to be a channel, that you want to surrender to the energy which strives to come through you, the faster will be your progress, and the sooner you will come into relationship with the All. In the *Bible* we read, "Call unto me, and I will answer thee, and show thee great and mighty things, which thou knowest not."[42]

Affirmations have their greatest effect when a person is in the alpha/theta state. Moreover, achieving the alpha/theta state is a prerequisite for success in all forms of healing. So we will begin our first healing meditation by entering the alpha/theta level.

Healing at the Alpha/Theta Level

To enter the alpha/theta level, simply follow these

directions; find a comfortable position with your back straight and begin the Yogic breathing you learned earlier, breathing fully without separation between inhalation and exhalation. Relax while you continue with the Yogic breathing, and begin slowly counting backwards from 5 to 1, repeating and visualizing each number three times to yourself. When you've reached the number 1, repeat to yourself, "I am now deeply relaxed, feeling better than I did before." Continue with deep Yogic breathing and when you're ready count backwards from 10 to 1, exhaling as you mentally repeat each number. Continue in this way until you've reached the number 1. By this time you should be feeling very light, very relaxed and wide-awake mentally. Now affirm to yourself, "Every time I come to this level of mind I learn to use more of my mind in more creative ways."

The Central Pranic Vibration

There is an alternative method for relaxing the physical body which you will learn in this meditation. Instead of tightening and releasing different parts of your physical body as you did during mental projection, in this meditation you will consciously pay attention to each part of your body, first stimulating it mentally and then feeling a vibration flowing through it. Then you will mentally experience all tension being released. The vibration I'm speaking of is called the "central pranic vibration." It is with you all the time. It is a manifestation of your etheric body. You become consciously aware of it whenever the etheric body is released from the confinement of the physical body. This can happen while you are in the alpha/theta level, during meditation as well as during sleep.

I know that some of you have awakened suddenly from sleep with your physical body vibrating so powerfully that you were unable to move it. This temporary vibration and paralysis will occur when a person regains consciousness before the etheric body has re-entered the glove of the physical body.

While you are asleep the etheric body moves outside the physical body where it is recharged by energy from the higher planes. This is one of the functions of sleep. If you are conscious while the etheric body is slightly outside the physical body or if you have integrated unconscious mental activity with conscious mental activity, you will consciously experience this vibration. The latter is exactly what happens while you are practicing healing in the alpha/theta level. While you are functioning at the alpha/theta level, you should pay attention and let yourself experience the renewing effects of the central pranic vibration. It is beneficial because it relaxes and renews the physical body and because it can be used in direct healing, with "laying on hands".

Relaxing the Physical Body

You begin relaxing your physical body by paying attention to your feet; if you pay attention to them for even a few moments, you will begin to feel them tingle. The tingling sensation is caused by circulation. It is not the pranic vibration, but will sometimes trigger it. Paying attention has the added feature of keeping you in the alpha/theta level. If you remain in this level long enough, you will begin to feel the pranic vibration. But for now, just pay attention to your toes, feel the tingling sensation in them and then feel your toes relax. Next feel the vibration spread through your feet and feel your feet relax. Continue the process by paying attention to your ankles. Pay attention to them until they begin to tingle and relax. You might find it helpful and relaxing to visualize yourself massaging or stroking your ankles. You can use this visualization with any part of your body you think it will benefit. Mentally talking to different parts of your body will help them relax. Remember that each cell has its own center of consciousness and both your thoughts and words influence them.

Continue the process of physical relaxation by bringing your attention to your calves. From there move to your knees. From your knees feel the tingling sensation move to your thighs. Pay attention to your thighs until they are completely relaxed. Continue in this way with your hips, your buttocks, pelvic region, lower abdomen and lower back, upper abdomen and middle back. Then pay attention to your breath and follow it until it gets deeper and more rhythmic. Visualize prana entering your respiratory system on each inhalation, and on each exhalation visualize prana in the form of a fluid bursting with energy, radiating through your chest. Then feel the tingling sensation in your chest and shoulders. Pay attention to your shoulders and feel them relax. By now some of you will feel the central pranic vibration. You will be able to distinguish the pranic vibration from other sensations and vibrations because only the pranic vibration continues after you have removed your attention from it. After you feel your shoulders relax, focus your attention on your fingers. Then continue the process of relaxation with your fingers, hands, wrists, lower arms, elbows, upper arms; then move to your neck. Your face gets special attention. Most people have emotional tensions stored in the muscles of their face. Start with the jaw, then go to your chin, mouth, cheeks, nose, ears, eyes, forehead; feel the tingling sensation move up the back of your neck and finally feel your entire scalp tingling and completely relaxed. By now most of you should feel the tingling sensation being replaced by the central pranic vibration. Usually the pranic vibration begins in the chest, but it will quickly radiate through the entire body if the body is completely relaxed.

For some of you it will take a little practice to recognize the central pranic vibration, and just about everyone needs practice in working with it. As soon as your entire body has been relaxed and you feel the central pranic vibration flowing through it, visualize and experience a wave of energy flowing into your crown chakra and from there feel it flowing from your crown chakra and into each part of your body. Feel the energy relax and revitalize your body. Then let your mind drift. As it drifts and spontaneous visual images begin appearing mentally affirm,

"Every time I come to this level of mind, it makes it easier for me to go into deeper and healthier levels of mind." Then visualize yourself in your sanctuary. Remain there for about five minutes or until you are satisfied. Then return from your sanctuary and mentally affirm, "I am an open channel for healing, and healing energy is flowing through me."

The Visual Screen

Next, visualize a white screen (like a movie screen), six feet in front of you. Visualize it on a platform, so that the screen reaches thirty degrees above your head. Mentally repeat the name of the person you want healed. Lift your gaze thirty degrees upward and you will see the person appear on your visual screen. This shouldn't require any effort if you are at the right level of consciousness. If you are in the alpha/theta level, your patient will spontaneously appear on the screen.Your patient will remain on the screen without wavering if you open your heart, the fourth chakra and reach out and hold him on the screen with love. I have found that nearly all problems in visualization are solved when the healer opens his heart and feels affection and compassion for the person he is visualizing on the screen. Once you see your patient on your screen, visualize yourself standing beside him rather than six feet away. Take your right hand and mentally place it on the diseased area of your patient's body and mentally place your left hand opposite it. (see plate) If your patient has a heart condition, for example, place your right hand on the heart and place your left hand on his back opposite it. Keep all five of your senses open, active and alert, and allow yourself to feel. Now, by feeling, I don't mean to become emotionally attached. In healing as in all spiritual and psychic work, you never turn off your senses and feelings. On the contrary, to become an effective channel you must allow your emotions to flow freely and you must keep your senses open. You simply avoid becoming caught up in the results or fruit of your work. You shouldn't let your ego get so

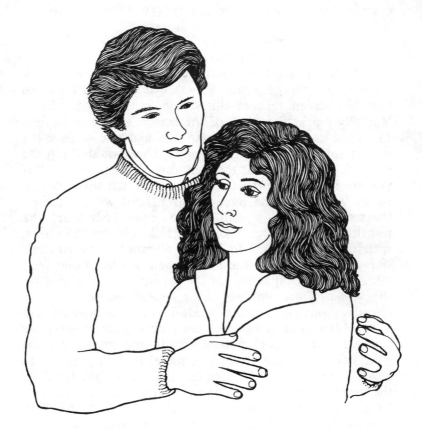

Plate 4: The Visual Screen

involved in your work that you become personally attached to the process. In healing, since you are only a channel, you must always do your work without thought of reward in mind. This attitude of "charity", as the New Testament describes it, is essential. The *Bhagavad Gita* explains, "In this world, people are fettered by action unless it is performed as sacrifice. Therefore . . . let thy acts be done without attachment, as sacrifice only."[43]

You must remember that if you want to hold your visualization without having it waver, you must open your heart and hold the image on your screen by paying attention to it with your heart and with your unconscious mind.

By applying mental attention to your heart, you activate it. By bringing your breath to your heart and placing your right hand on it, emotions of love will be activated and by directing this energy to your patient you should have no problem with mental visualization. Once you've visualized your hands on your patient, imagine that your hands are becoming hot and that energy is flowing through them. It is important to empathize as much as possible with your patient, because in the next step, you must feel him absorbing the energy. You must feel him accept it gratefully and if possible, you should allow yourself to feel the positive effects the energy is having upon him as it flows into his body. Take your time and let yourself become immersed in this part of the healing process; experience it in its fullness. The less you think of yourself and the more you apply yourself to what you are doing, the better, so be patient and allow the healing energy to flow through you. I suggest that in the beginning you spend about five minutes practicing this particular visualization.

Recharging the Aura
Once you feel satisfied this procedure has benefited your patient, visualize yourself six feet in front of the visual screen again. Then, take a deep breath and feel yourself going deeper. Feel energy surging through your hands

again, but instead of projecting it to one specific part of your patient's body, fill your patient's aura (the energy field around him) with healing energy. This visualization is easiest to do if you imagine rays of light flowing from your hands and filling the patient's aura with light. As you send these rays of energy, visualize your patient smiling, happy and healthy, remembering that what you create on the mental plane will sooner or later be transmuted to the physical plane. Continue filling his aura with energy, and again, feel him absorb it, but this time as warmth which radiates through his skin into each part of his body, down to the cells themselves. In the beginning, I suggest you spend about two to three minutes with this technique. It will have a strong, positive effect on your patient. It recharges him, filling him with energy (prana). It increases his vitality which is especially useful when you have a patient who is run down. Your patient absorbs the prana you transmit and he is recharged by it, in the same way a car battery is recharged when you give it a boost from another fully charged battery. You shouldn't dismiss this technique lightly since the healer never directly affects the patient's physical body. The healer works on the higher planes and the patient ends up healing himself by transmuting the energy coming through the healer. The healer can only affect the patient's etheric and mental bodies. It's up to the patient to allow the energy to become effective on the physical plane. That is why the patient's attitude is so important. The more receptive the patient is, the more benefit he will derive from spiritual healing. In the final analysis, it is always the patient who heals himself. Any technique which channels prana to the patient and fills his aura with energy will be useful in the healing process, because if the patient is receptive, he will permit the energy flowing into his subtle energy system (which exists on the etheric plane) to be transmuted to the physical plane. There, it can be used to heal physical disease.

   In the beginning, take between three and five minutes

to fill your patient's aura with healing energy. When his aura is fully charged, it should glow with vitality, it should increase in size and the texture should become smooth and uniform throughout its entire surface. Any dark patches that appeared in the aura prior to recharging should have disappeared by now. When you feel satisfied that your patient's aura is fully charged, then take a deep inhalation and relax, and as you relax, mentally affirm, "God has healed you, is healing you and will continue to heal you." Then release your patient, take another deep breath and on the exhalation, release the screen.

Recharging the "Subtle Energy System"

In the final stage of a healing meditation, the healer always takes time to recharge himself. Begin recharging by taking a deep breath, holding it for a moment, and as you do, let your mind drift. As it drifts, feel a wave of energy flowing through the top of your head (crown chakra) and feel it flow through your entire body, refreshing it and healing it. Feel it exit through your finger tips and toes, and as it does, feel another wave of energy take its place. Feel one wave after another pass through your body until you feel your chakras glowing. At first, the glowing sensation might be subtle and might be confined to the crown chakra, but the more healing you do the more powerful the sensation will become.

As Divine energy flows through a person, it affects the energy centers (chakras). In time, as all the chakras are opened and balanced, the energy radiates through all the chakras at once. Each chakra will produce its own characteristic sensations. These sensations are positive signs since they indicate that the chakras are open and healing energy is passing through them. Having these experiences has in many spiritual traditions been considered a gift from God, so I encourage you to experience these sensations fully when they occur.

You should intuitively choose the amount of time you need for recharging. When I do direct healing (laying on of hands), I usually take between three and five minutes. When I do absentee healing during my own meditations, I often take considerably longer.

The final steps of this meditation, as well as the meditations I will discuss later, involve the return trip to normal consciousness. You always begin your return to normal consciousness with an affirmation. After you feel fully recharged, mentally affirm, "Every time I channel healing energy, I am also healed and I become a more powerful channel for healing." Then slowly begin counting from 1 to 5. Count 1, 2, then say to yourself, "I am coming up slowly . . . count 3, 4, 5 . . . then open your eyes. When you reach 5 say to yourself, "I feel wide awake, perfectly relaxed, and better than I did before.

CHAPTER NINE

MENTAL HEALING

As you know, a person can project his consciousness (his unconscious mind) anywhere in the universe he wants. It is an ability which lies dormant in everyone and it is an essential part of absentee healing. You began mastering the technique earlier, in mental projection and in the visual screen. In this chapter you will take this technique a step further by projecting your consciousness into the physical body of another person and performing a healing while you are inside. You should begin this technique by finding a comfortable position, preferably with your back straight. Then close your eyes and begin breathing deeply, without separation between inhalation and exhalation. After breathing in this way for a few moments, you will enter the alpha/theta level. While at this level, not only can you project your consciousness into another person's body, you can serve as a channel for his healing.

Continue by breathing Yogically for two or three minutes and then start counting backwards from 5 to 1. On every descending number repeat and visualize each number three times to yourself. Take your time. When you feel ready, mentally affirm, "I am now in the alpha state, feeling better than I did before." Continue to breathe deeply, and after a few moments, slowly begin counting backwards from 10 to 1; mentally repeating each number as you exhale, continuing in this manner until you reach the number 1. After you reach the number 1, repeat this second affirmation to yourself, "Every time I come to this level of mind, it makes it easier for me to go to deeper and healthier levels." Then pay attention to your feet. In a few moments you will feel a vibration in your feet. Feel the vibration move through your feet, relaxing the muscles, bones and tissues completely. Follow the vibration as it moves through your feet into your ankles. Feel your ankles relax as all stress and tension is released. Continue to follow the vibration as it moves through your calves, relaxing them as well. Then pay attention as the vibration moves into each part of your physical body. Feel each part vibrate, as all stress and tension is released. As the vibration reaches each part of your body, repeat this affirmation, "I feel the vibration and my (insert part of body) is completely re-laxed." This will cue the centers of consciousness through-out your physical body, and they will relax completely.

When you feel your entire body vibrating and all stress and tension gone, mentally affirm, "My body is completely relaxed, feeling better than it did before." Then allow your mind to drift, and after a few moments visualize yourself in your sanctuary. Give yourself about five minutes to enjoy your sanctuary, during which time you should feel the central pranic vibration as it radiates through your body. After about five minutes mentally return to your meditation place and affirm to yourself, "I am an open channel, and healing energy is flowing through me. Then visualize your visual screen two meters in front of you, rising above your head thirty degrees. Mentally repeat the name of the person you want to heal, then lift your eyes thirty degrees and you will see the person appear on your screen.

Using the Third Chakra

In the last chapter, you performed an absentee healing while outside your patient's body, using the fourth and sixth chakras. To work inside your patient's physical body, you must pay attention to your third chakra (solar plexus) and work from it as well. To work inside your patient's body, begin by paying attention and breathing from your heart chakra. After a few moments put your hand on your heart to hold your patient on your visual screen more easily. Scan his body for a few moments and empathize with him until you feel his "essential" qualities and vibration. Empathizing with him is important in establishing a rapport and feeling him in his fullness. Next, pay attention to your third chakra, while holding your patient in front of you with love. Continue paying attention to your third chakra, until you feel it vibrating. When you feel the vibration, imagine a cord stretching from your solar plexus to the solar plexus of your patient. Then feel yourself being pulled towards your patient, and feel the tug come from the cord which now links you together. Don't resist, rather allow yourself to be pulled into your patient, as the cord between you gets shorter. You will finally experience yourself merging with your patient as you surrender completely.

Diagnosis Inside the Body

By using the third chakra in this way, you will make deeper contact with your patient and you will be able to sense his feelings and the negative vibrations in his subtle energy system more easily. When you are inside your patient's body, mentally affirm, "I am standing between my patient's lungs". Instantaneously you will be there in the appropriate size to fit comfortably. Reach out your hand and touch one of his lungs; use all of your senses to examine the lung completely. Feel the "rightness" or "wrongness" of his lung; feel any "wobbles" in its vibration. Take two or three minutes to examine one lung, then the other. When you are finished, take a deep breath and as you exhale, visualize yourself standing by his spine. Examine the spine and the tissue surrounding it for two or three minutes. Notice the differences between the various tissues. When you are satisfied that you have experienced the spinal area in its fullness, take a deep breath and visualize yourself standing by the diseased area of your patient's body. If, for example, the kidney is diseased, then imagine you are standing next to the diseased kidney. Once you are beside the damaged organ you will see a difference between the diseased tissue and the healthy tissue you observed before. Feel the "wobbles" in its vibration; check the texture, temperature and finally color. Diseased tissue is usually dark in color and has an irregular texture and shape. Often the tissue will look lumpy, or feel too cold or too hot. If you see brown, black, grey, muddy yellow or muddy green; if you see any dirty, muddy colors at all, you will know there is a problem in the area. Diagnosing what is wrong on the etheric and mental levels will help you by providing insight into which healing technique will be most effective.

Healing Inside the Body

Once you've examined the diseased tissue, mentally place your hands on it and feel energy flowing from your hands into it. The hands should be opposite each other and should not be touching. Feel energy flowing through your hands and feel them get hot. Then feel your patient absorb the energy flowing into them, with gratitude. Send your patient healing energy in this way for two or three minutes. Then imagine yourself with a set of tools which you can use for healing; doctor's tools, kitchen tools, mechanic's tools, painter's tools. In absentee healing any tools will do, even tools like ray guns, etc. which you invent yourself. Then take five minutes to heal your patient using your tools.

Healing Visualizations

I use tools whenever I perform an absentee healing. Below are two visualizations using tools which have proven effective for me. In the first, I worked on a patient who suffered a broken leg while skiing in Colorado. I was unable to see him in person, so all the work was done at a distance. I began the healing by visualizing myself inside his body, standing beside the fracture. I brought glue with me and visualized myself applying it to both ends of the broken bone. I waited a moment and then squeezed the two ends together. I held them together until the glue set and the bone was firmly reconnected. Then I mixed a plaster compound and I applied it to the seam where I had connected the two bones. I waited for it to harden, then took a file and sanded the area to make it perfectly smooth. Finally, I squeezed out medicine from a tube labeled "healing medicine". I applied it to the crack and then ran my hands over the crack, rubbing the medicine in; all the time imagining healing energy flowing from my hands into the bone, healing it completely. The reports I received later comfirmed that the bone healed in record time.

In the other case, I worked on a baby who had fallen down a flight of stairs. When I was asked to work on her, she was in critical condition. The child had torn ligaments in the back of her neck and was bleeding internally, and had multiple blood clots in the arteries and veins of her neck and head. In this case, I repeated the procedures below on the damaged veins, arteries and ligaments. First, I visualized myself in the baby's neck, standing within one of the clogged vessels. I visualized myself with an electric drill and began using it to break up the blood clots in her neck. When the clots were broken up into small pieces, I visualized myself sweeping them up and putting them into a bucket I had with me. I went from one blood vessel to the next until all were unclogged. Then I began working on the torn ligaments and muscles. I repaired them by sewing the ripped ends together. I imagined that I had a needle and thread with me, and sewed together each ligament and each torn muscle. Finally, I returned to the blood vessels and applied "healing medicine" to the ones I had repaired. I did the same with the muscles and ligaments, applying medicine to each one I had sewn back together. This procedure took me more than four hours, but it was well worth it, because the next day I was informed the baby was out of danger and was making a rapid recovery.

Using Your Tools

When you practice mental healing, take about five minutes to heal with your tools. Become as creative as you like. It's often a good idea during mental healing to mentally talk to your patient. I encourage my patients, by telling them that energy is flowing through them and the energy is healing them. As I speak I imagine my patients absorbing the energy, and I feel it healing them. Sometimes my patients respond mentally, telling me where they are blocked or where they need more energy. These mental conversations help me feel more deeply for them. When I feel more, my chakras are open wider and more energy flows through them. As a result, my patients and I come into closer rapport. So feel free to express yourself while you are within your patient's body, especially while you are working on the diseased tissue with your tools.

Recharging Your Patient's Aura

After you have finished working with your tools and the diseased area looks completely healed, visualize yourself outside your patient's body, six feet in front of the screen. Take a deep breath and feel yourself going deeper. Then feel energy surge through your hands. Visualize the energy flowing through your hands into your patient's aura. Visualize the energy as luminous rays flowing from your hands, filling your patient's aura with light. As he absorbs the energy from your hands, visualize him smiling, happy and in perfect health. While he is smiling, see him absorb the energy through his skin and feel it revitalize every cell in his body.Continue for two or three minutes, then release the rays of energy from your hands and visualize your hands at your sides again. Release your patient and your visual screen. Then take a deep breath and relax.

Recharging Yourself

Next recharge yourself by imagining a wave of energy flowing into your crown chakra. Feel it flow from the crown chakra into every part of your body, recharging every cell. Continue recharging until you feel all of your chakras glowing.

Begin your return trip to outer consciousness by mentally affirming, "Every time I do healing, I am healed and I become a more powerful channel for healing." Then count from 1 to 5 slowly, and when you reach the number 5, open your eyes. You will feel wide awake, perfectly relaxed and better than you did before.

Dr. Simington and Mental Healing

Dr. Carl Simington and his wife, Stephanie, are leaders in the field of holistic health, and have been using visualization and relaxation in their treatment of cancer since the early 1970's, and their results have been well documented. The startling fact is that the survival rate of the Simington's patients are currently twice the national norm in the United States. Below is a summary of results they had with a group of cancer patients who before the Simingtons began treating them were pronounced incurable by the traditional medical community. None of them were given more than one year to live, prior to beginning treatment with the Simingtons. These patients were each treated by the Simingtons for a minimum of four years from 1974–1978. Of 159 patients, from whom this data is drawn in 1978, 63 were still alive. Of these, 22.2% or 14 patients showed no evidence of disease; 19.1% or 12 patients showed that tumors were regressing; 27.1% or 17 patients showed the cancer stable and 31.8% or 20 patients showed no tumor growth.

A Case History

Below is a dramatic case history that impressed the Simingtons in the beginning of their work. It occurred in 1971, when a man who had a type of throat cancer came to them for treatment. He was in grave condition and there was little chance that he would recover. He had already lost a considerable amount of weight and he was in an extremely weakened condition when he arrived. Before his cancer developed he weighed 130 pounds, but he had lost 32 pounds and at the time weighed 98 pounds. Even worse, he could barely swallow his own saliva and was having difficulty breathing. His diagnosis was clear; he had less than a 5% chance of living for more than five years. He had been treated by the staff of a well-known medical school and the physicians there were unsure if continued treatment was advisable since they considered his case hopeless. They believed treatment would only make him more miserable, without necessarily helping his condition.

Dr. Simington began treating the patient by explaining that success depended on the patient's active participation in the treatment. He explained to the patient that he himself had the power to influence the course of his own disease. He then devised a program of relaxation, affirmation and visualization. The patient was told that three times daily he must set aside periods of between five and fifteen minutes for self-healing: when he woke up in the morning, after lunch, and at night before going to bed. During these periods he was instructed to sit quietly and relax. He was told to begin his relaxation by paying attention to the muscles of his body and mentally telling each group of muscles to relax. Once he was in the alpha/theta level, he was to go to a place where he was perfectly relaxed, where he was at perfect peace. After he returned from his perfect place of relaxation, he was asked to visualize his cancer clearly, in whatever form it took.

Next, Dr. Simington instructed the man to visualize the radiation treatment he was undergoing as consisting of millions of little energy projectiles which bombarded the cancerous cells in their path. Since the normal cells were stronger and healthier than the cancerous cells, the projectiles wouldn't harm them, but the weaker cancer cells would be damaged beyond repair and they would die. In the final stage of this treatment, the patient was asked to visualize his body's white blood cells swarming over the cancer cells, collecting the dead and dying ones and then carrying them off to the liver and kidneys where they would be flushed out of his body. Then he was told to see his cancer shrinking in size in each successive meditation, until the cancer disappeared and his body returned to normal. The results of combined radiation and visualization treatments went beyond anything the Simingtons expected, or anything they had previously experienced in purely physical intervention. The patient made remarkable progress; he showed virtually no ill effects from the radiation treatment. Halfway through the treatment his throat was so improved he could eat again. He gained weight and strength and his general appearance showed a remarkable improvement. But what was most important, his cancer progressively disappeared.

An important element of the Simington's treatment was instilling in their patient a sense of control over his body and over the course of his disease. In the case just cited, the patient reported missing only one session of visualization during his course of treatment and interestingly, he told the Simingtons that he was quite upset about missing it because he felt by missing the session he was losing control over his treatment and it could weaken his ability to influence his state of health.The patient continued his rapid progress under the Simington's care and within two months after beginning treatment, there were no longer any signs of cancer. His firm belief that he could influence the course of his disease was made most evident when near the end of his treatment he said to Carl Simington, "Doctor, in the beginning I needed you in order to get well, Now I think you could disappear and I could still make it on my own."[44]

CHAPTER TEN

HEALING DIAGNOSIS AND THE AURA

I spoke earlier about the organs or the "subtle energy system," and in particular, the chakras. The chakras channel prana, the absolute energy, from the higher planes into the human aura. Each chakra channels different frequencies of prana into a person's aura, and like the visual spectrum of light, these frequencies can be broken down into different colors. These colors are visible to the trained healer, and they provide him with a picture of his patient's state of health.

The Three Auras
Every human being has three auras; a spiritual aura, a mental aura and an etheric aura. The highest frequencies of prana are confined to the spiritual aura. But prana is also transmuted into mental energy and this form of energy appears in the mental aura. Other energy is transmuted further into etheric energy, and this energy as well as energy from the physical body is confined to the etheric aura.

The spiritual aura extends the farthest from the physical body. It has a radius of about twenty five feet in a healthy human being. Within it is the mental aura, which is composed of energy from the mental body. The energy from it extends about eight feet in a normal human being, and it reflects the mental state of a person. The final aura reflects the emotional and physical health of a person. It is called the etheric aura. It extends about eight inches from the physical body.

In healing we are primarily concerned with the etheric aura because when disease is present in either the etheric body or the physical body, it disrupts the subtle energy system, and healthy frequencies are transmuted into unhealthy ones. With a shift in frequency, there is a shift in color in the patient's etheric aura. The healer can see when the normal colors indicating good health become muddy, dirty, or change from bright, clear primary colors associated with good health, to earth tones; browns, greys, and black, all of which are associated with disease.

In *The Power of the Rays*, S. G. J. Ouseley tells us "The aura is the expression of the real man . . . It is the sum total of his forces and emotions—physical, etheric, astral, mental and spiritual. Concisely speaking, it is a subtle super-physical emanation surrounding a person in the form of a luminous mist or cloud. The auric emanation is the essence of a man's life—it reveals his character, emotional nature, mental calibre, state of health and spiritual development."[45]

By examining the colors and qualities of his patient's aura, a healer can tell the nature and severity of his patient's disease and he can determine the kind of energy his patient needs to regain his health and balance. Then, the healer can project the necessary healing energy, in the appropriate color, to his patient.

There are three ways a healer can see his patient's aura: the healer can see the aura by developing his auric vision, the healer can feel the aura through the palms of his hands, and finally, the healer can see the aura clairvoyantly.

The Aura and Dr. Kilner

The English scientist Walter J. Kilner pioneered scientific research into the human aura. In 1908 Kilner came up with the idea that the aura could be made visible if viewed through a screen coated with a suitable dye. He experimented with Dicyanin, a coal tar derivative and found it had an extraordinary effect on the eyesight. He discovered the coal tar produced a temporary shortsightedness when people gazed through a screen coated with it. When they looked through it people became more sensitive to radiation from the ultraviolet end of the spectrum. For some reason, this increased sensitivity allowed people to see the etheric aura clearly. Kilner also found that the aura was more visible when light was shaded, and he conducted most of his experiments in semi-darkened rooms. He discovered that a black background improved auric vision, therefore, in many of his experiments he placed a subject in a darkened room about ten inches from a dark wall and then examined the person through the Dicyanin screen.

In later years it was discovered that the screen could be discarded because it was the temporary shortsightedness which was the important factor in seeing the aura. Shortsightedness can be easily achieved by simply looking past an object until the eyes unfocus.

Seeing the Aura

Later researchers found that four conditions must be met in order to physically see the etheric aura. First, the observer must be in the alpha/theta level. Second, the heart chakra must be open. Third, the room must be darkened, and a dark background must be behind the person being viewed. Lastly, the observer must allow his eyes to unfocus without straining them.

The aura is most readily seen around the head, hands and feet. You should begin looking for the aura around your hands. To see the aura around your hands, you will need a black piece of cardboard about three feet long and eighteen inches wide. To begin, sit upright with your back straight and start breathing Yogically. Continue with the yogic breath for two or three minutes and then begin a short meditation. At first, meditate for at least ten minutes using the techniques you've already learned. This will bring you firmly into the alpha/theta state, and you will be thinking in pictures rather than words. I suggest that after you have counted backwards from 5 to 1; 10 to 1, and after you have relaxed your body completely, you go to your sanctuary and remain there for five minutes. When you return from there, mentally affirm, "I am perfectly relaxed, feeling better than I did before, and I am able to see the aura." Then count from 1 to 5, and when you open your eyes, look down past your hands into the cardboard below them. For best results your hands should be held three inches above the cardboard in a horizontal position, palms up with the fingers pointing towards each other and almost touching. The fingers should be comfortably spread out. Once you've begun looking past your hands and through your fingers, your eyes will unfocus without any difficulty. Bring your attention to the heart chakra and begin breathing from it, and you will see the aura appear between your fingers. (See plate)

At first, the aura may be faint and difficult to see; it might look something like steam evaporating, but if you continue relaxing, going deeper, paying attention without concentrating, the aura will get brighter. As the brightness grows stronger, colors will begin to emerge. When this happens, slowly spread your hands apart and you will see lines of force connecting your fingers. These lines will connect the corresponding fingers of each hand and will join them together, until you've spread the hands six or eight inches apart. Then the lines will split down the center, and you will see the aura surrounding each hand separately. After you have mastered this technique, it will become progressively easier for you to see the colors around your hands. When you feel confident of your ability, begin examining the auras of your friends and associates. The auras around their heads will be easiest for you to see. You need only observe them while you are relaxed (in the alpha/theta state) with your heart chakra open, and when they have a clear, darkened background behind them.

When you want to see another person's aura, use one of the methods you learned earlier to put yourself in the alpha/theta state. Then, unfocus your eyes and look past him into the clear background. The aura around the head

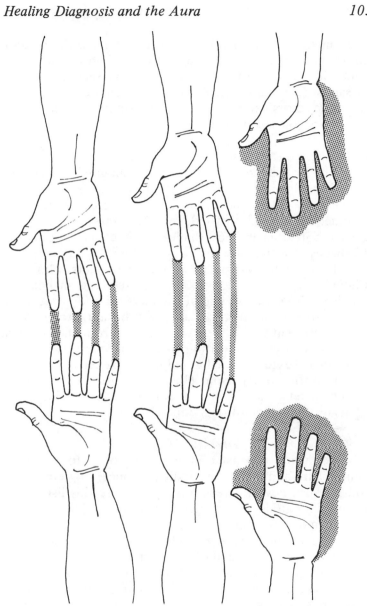

Plate 5: Seeing the Aura

will emerge first as a mist, then in colors, with the dark colors emerging first, followed by the lighter ones. The aura will resemble the halos which you've seen in portraits of saints. (See plate) Once you've mastered the technique, the auric colors will become as bright or even brighter than the colors you see in the material world.

The Aura's Features

The British Color Council has catalogued auric colors and found an astonishing number of colors within the human aura. To this date, they have discovered 1,400 shades of blue, 1,000 shades of red, over 1,400 browns, over 800 greens, 550 oranges, 360 shades of violet, and more than 12 shades of white.

It is generally agreed among researchers who have studied the aura that it is more or less egg shaped and usually follows the outline of the physical body, but it can vary. People with greater vitality will have a stronger aura and consequently it will extend further from the physical body. Also, the composition of the aura varies with each individual. Texture as well as color and size seem to indicate the disposition of a person. The texture often tells us about the character of a person, while the shape and color shows us his health and emotional condition.

The Auric Colors

Following is a list of the major colors found in the human aura and what they indicate concerning emotional and physical health. I recommend you use this list simply as an initial guide. Later, make up your own list based on your own observations.

You should note that within the etheric aura there is sometimes a narrow band of uniform color surrounding the physical body. It usually looks dark or colorless and often appears as a gap between the physical body and the etheric aura. It is not seen around everyone, but for those who have it, it doesn't appear to affect them in a negative way. It is an interesting anomaly which for convenience's sake is

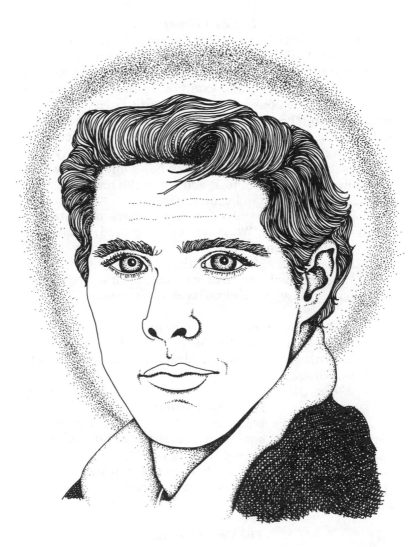

Plate 6: The Aura Around the Head

called the physical aura.

The Red Group

In the etheric aura, the red group of colors have the lowest visible vibration. They have a dual nature; in their positive form when they are bright and clear, their aspects are energizing, warming and exciting. Their negative aspects range from rebelliousness and contentiousness to anger, malice, destructiveness and hate. When the red is very dark, it indicates selfishness and lack of nobility. A deep red usually indicates passion. When it becomes muddy, the passions become unclean and unwholesome. Red which has brown in it indicates fear, and when the brown darkens and becomes black, it indicates malice.

When red has a tint of yellow, we see uncontrolled emotions and desires. When we see a light red, it indicates a nervous temperament and a bright, clear red shows vitality, generosity and material health. A rosy brightness shows filial affection and the love of home, while red which moves into pink shows happiness and tenderness.

The Orange Group

Orange in its clearest form indicates forcefulness and vitality. When it becomes reddish, it tends to indicate self-centeredness.

The Yellow Group

Yellow is the color of intellect. When it is dull, it indicates intellect, but of a mundane nature. When it becomes brighter, moving into gold, there is an elevation of the intellect and it becomes purified through spirit. Muddy or dirty yellow indicates cunning, greed and self-centered egotism.

The Green Group

Green is the color of balance. It is the color of the heart. Emerald green, which is clear and bright, is the color of healing. A great deal of emerald green in a person's

aura indicates an interest or involvement in the healing arts.
Green is the central color in the spectrum of light. It
is midway between the extremes of red and violet, and
when we see it in a person's aura, it indicates balance,
harmony and flexibility. Light green indicates harmony,
peacefulness and an affinity to nature and the outdoors. In
its negative form, green indicates extreme selfishness.
When it is muddy and dirty, it shows deceitfulness and
greed. When it becomes brownish, it indicates jealousy.

The Blue Group

The blue color has always been associated with religious feelings and intuitive understanding. Just as green is
associated with healing and the heart, blue in its highest
form is associated with the Third Eye, inspiration and the
higher forms of intellect. It is one of the first colors a
healer sees. Ouseley calls blue, "heaven's own color"[46] and
associates it with loftiest spiritual aspirations and with the
feminine aspect of nature, the subjective intuitive mind.
When blue deepens into indigo, we find a person with a
devotional character and a deeply religious spirit. On the
negative side, blue with brown or black in it shows a per-
version of religious feelings, indicating a fascination with
the darker side of spirituality.

The Violet Group

Violet, which is a combination of red and blue, points
to even loftier spiritual ideals and power. Those who have
violet in their aura have advanced farthest in their spiritual
evolution. It is the color of royalty and indicates nobility
of character. Violet in the aura acts as an insulator and
purifier. It is not a common color in the average aura. It
is a color that comes from the higher realms and thus is
seen only in spiritual masters and adepts. When it shades
into lavender, it denotes high spirituality as well as vitality.
When it shades into lilac, it shows a compassionate and
altruistic character.
Violet first appears above the head and looks like an

ovoid atop the crown chakra. As the adept advances, the violet radiates from there, filling the entire aura with its light.

The Brown Group
Brown is a combination of all colors but is not itself a color found in the spectrum. Some researchers connect brown with business and industry, calling it the business man's color. But I have generally found that it has a negative influence in the aura, being the color most often associated with physical disease. Most healers associate brown with negative human characteristics. In its various forms, it indicates stinginess, greed and the lower material instincts. Only when it becomes a golden brown does its vibration rise, showing an industrious, organized character and a methodical temperament.

Black
Black, which is the absence of light, indicates darkness on all levels. The only exception is when it appears in a narrow band often seen between the physical body and the etheric aura, what we call the physical aura. Black, when it fills the aura indicates the negation of life itself; when streaks of black are seen within an otherwise normal aura, the effect of the streaks is unfortunate, since they neutralize the good aspects in the aura.

The Gray Group
Gray is also a negative color, showing a dull, conventional character. It indicates dullness on the physical level, and shows a lack of vitality, which is often associated with disease. Heavy, deep grays indicate fear, confusion and often a dull, heavy, leaden personality often bordering on morbidity. Gray in the aura often indicates an unreliable, deceptive character.

White
Finally, we come to white, which is the synthesis of

all colors, indicating complete integration and the capacity for union. It is the color of Christ Consciousness, the color of the I AM. It is the color of spiritual perfection and is found only in those who have achieved union and who have attained enlightenment.

Feeling the Aura

Each of us has the capacity to feel the etheric aura, as well as to see it. Feeling the surface of the etheric aura is a common method of psychic diagnosis. We can tell a great deal about a person's aura, not only by the colors, but by its shape, texture and strength. The healer, by stroking the surface of his patient's aura with the palm of his hand, can collect information about the physical health and emotional well-being of his patient. Stroking the surface of the etheric aura is a simple technique, and if you follow the accompanying directions, you should be able to use it successfully.

You should begin practicing the technique of feeling the aura by having your patient lie down on his back. It is important for your patient to be as relaxed as possible. If he doesn't meditate or do spiritual exercises, I suggest you lead him into the three part Yogic breathing. Have him continue with the Yogic breathing for two or three minutes. Since changes can occur in your patient's aura as a result of strong feelings, excitement or anxiety, having your patient relaxed is essential for receiving accurate impressions. When he is relaxed, use the techniques you learned earlier to put yourself in the alpha/theta level. Once you have entered the alpha/theta level, mentally affirm, "I am now in the alpha level and my hands are becoming sensitive." Then make three complete passes with your hands over your subject's body, starting at his head and ending at his feet. These passes should be made with both hands about eight inches above your patient's body, palms down, with fingers loosely extended. Hands should not be touching. After the final pass, have your patient close his eyes and place your more sensitive hand about eighteen inches above his heart. Let your hand descend until you feel a slight resistance, which will make the palm of your hand tingle. The resistance comes from the surface of your patient's aura. As we know, the etheric aura extends about eight inches from the physical body, and although it is fluid and porous throughout, it does have a skin-like surface. It can be likened to water, which has a distinct surface with distinct properties, but which can be passed through with ease.

Begin skimming the surface of your patient's aura, remaining attentive to the sensations in your palm. Always keep your palm on the surface. Only then will you receive accurate impressions of the aura's strength and texture. If you allow your hand to pass through the surface, you will feel the energy of your own hand as it is reflected from your patient's body. If you get close enough to his physical body, you will feel the heat generated by his body and nothing more. Skim the entire surface of your patient's aura and notice the sensations in your palm. Become aware of any changes in the aura's energy level which causes your hand to dip towards your patient's body or to be pushed farther away from it. Sharp changes signify problems in your patient's auric field and subtle energy system. Note differences in temperature; cold spots and warm spots can indicate the presence of disease as well.

The aura should be firm, smooth and of a uniform temperature. Whenever these conditions are altered, disease of some sort is the culprit. After you've registered all the impressions from the front of your patient's body, have him turn over and continue the procedure on his back. In the beginning be sure to get feedback from your subject. With practice you will become more sensitive and more confident, and you will recognize the sensations associated with different diseases and conditions. (See plate)

It might help you to keep a notebook and catalogue your findings. Every disease gives off a specific vibration and if you work intuitively, you will learn to discern the subtle distinctions of different diseases.

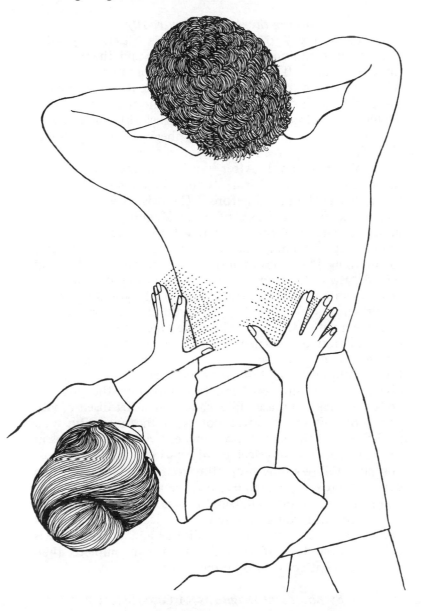

Plate 7: Feeling the Aura

Seeing the Aura Clairvoyantly

The third way to see the aura is to see it clairvoyantly. This is the technique I use most often and there are no limitations to it. It can be used at any time or any place, whether you are with your patient or not. It can be used in association with other psychic diagnostic techniques, so it should be developed by anyone who is working as a healer.

To see the aura clairvoyantly, begin breathing Yogically. Then use the techniques you learned earlier to enter the alpha/theta level. After you've returned from your sanctuary, mentally affirm, "I am now in the alpha level, feeling better than I did before." Then visualize your visual screen six feet in front of you. Mentally repeat your patient's name and your patient will then appear on your screen. Begin scanning your patient's body, being attentive to anything that doesn't look right. Problems will stand out; they will draw your attention. You might be looking at the aura around his head and suddenly you'll be drawn to his knee. When that happens, you can be sure there is a problem with the knee. Take some time then and examine the aura around the knee. Look at the color, texture and strength of it. Then go inside the physical body and look for any physical manifestations of disease. Find out if the disease in the aura has been transmuted to the physical body. In major diseases like cancer or heart disease, you will probably see negative colors in the aura. But you might not see the connection between various problems in the aura and the physical manifestation. If this happens, you must follow-up by projecting your consciousness inside your patient's physical body. For example, in heart disease you might see muddy colors in the aura above your patient's chest, but until you go inside the physical body you won't know the exact nature of the disease and your diagnosis will be incomplete. If your diagnosis is incomplete, then your treatment could also be incomplete.

Symbols and Diagnosis—A Case History

Sometimes even though you see problems in your

patient's aura, they show up symbolically rather than
objectively in the physical body. Here is a good example.
I was doing case readings with a friend. Case readings are
the best way I know for practicing psychic diagnosis. My
friend wrote the name, age and address of someone she
knew on the outside of a folded piece of paper. On the
inside she wrote down all the subject's medical and psychological problems. Since the paper was folded, I couldn't see
what was written on the inside. Then she guided me into a
short meditation similar to the one we use. After she guided
me back from my sanctuary, she told me the subject's
name, age and address, and then I saw the person appear
on my "visual screen".

I began scanning the body of a young woman, first
looking at her aura and then her physical body. I saw that
she was blonde, a little plump, and her cheeks were full
and rosy. She had a very broad smile on her face. I continued
looking, scanning her aura and physical body as far as her
shoulders, when I was quite suddenly drawn to her abdomen. I saw it was distended but I saw no problem in her
aura above the abdomen. When I projected my consciousness inside her abdomen, to my surprise I saw a basketball.
I was shocked, since I had never encountered anything like
it before. My first thought was that she had a tumor, but it
didn't feel right to me. She was so healthy looking and her
aura was primarily bright orange and golden yellow with
no unusual colors showing above her abdomen. Besides,
she was smiling and if I had a tumor the size of a basketball
in my abdomen, I don't think I would be smiling. Of course,
I finally saw I was being tricked; the woman wasn't sick at
all, she was pregnant. From then on, basketballs have
become my symbol for pregnancy.

Over the years I've evolved other symbols (and I
always use auric diagnosis in connection with them).
Varicose veins always look like strings, anemia looks like
diluted blood, arthritis looks like snowflakes resting on
bones, and ulcers are volcanoes erupting. Your symbols
may differ, but with experience you will discover their

meaning and will be able to use them effectively in diagnosis.

Clairsentience and Diagnosis

Not only can you see disease in your patient's aura, but you can often feel your patient's disease. The ability to do this is called clairsentience. Most psychics and healers have it. It is important for healers to develop clairsentience because it shows an empathetic nature which is important in healing. Your body is an instrument which will register discomforts from another person's body when you attune yourself to his vibration. So, expect to feel unusual sensations in your own body when you do diagnosis. Your "subtle energy system" will be receiving data from your patient and it will register the information as feelings, sensations and minor discomforts. These discomforts are temporary. They will have no lasting effect. It is a form of psychic communication which you should pay attention to and learn to use for diagnosis.

The aura, as you can see, is visible clairvoyantly. It can be felt with the palm, it can be seen physically, or it can be felt clairsentiently. Diagnosing from the aura should be a part of your psychic diagnosis. As you scan your patient's body, always look at his aura. Direct your attention to changes in the color, texture and size of your patient's aura. Use your auric vision along with your clairvoyance and clairsentience. They go hand in hand and most healers I know use these methods in combination for psychic diagnosis.

CHAPTER ELEVEN

CHAKRA HEALING

The "subtle energy system" brings energy from the higher planes into the physical body. When the subtle energy system acts as the recipient of energy, it is functioning in its feminine role, and by being receptive it has a negative polarization. As we know from the Hermetic philosophy, everything in the universe is polar, everything has its masculine and feminine, assertive and receptive aspects. So far you have learned about the feminine aspect of your subtle energy system, how it behaves in its receptive role. But the masculine aspect is just as important to the healer.

In this chapter you will learn about the masculine aspect of your subtle energy system, because even though the healer's subtle energy system receives healing energy from the higher planes, by becoming receptive, the healer channels energy through his subtle energy system to his patient by being assertive.

In spiritual healing the dual nature of your subtle energy system can be integrated in a technique called "chakra healing". In chakra healing, the healer takes in energy from the higher planes and channels the same energy through his chakras to his patient by projecting rays of energy to him. In this form of healing, energy is projected exclusively from the heart chakra and the third eye. The energy can be projected either as clear rays or colored rays; the colors fine-tune the healing energy by changing its vibration, providing the patient with the exact dosage of

115

energy he needs. Although you will be projecting rays of energy to your patient from the heart chakra and the third eye, it is important for you to keep all your chakras open during healing, because prana from all of them is being transmuted and used during a healing session. It is important to keep your crown chakra open during the healing process because the most profound healing energy enters your subtle energy system through your crown chakra.

Healing Rays and Emotions

We will begin chakra healing by projecting energy through our chakras as clear rays. Then we will send them in the appropriate healing colors. In chakra healing the healer is working directly from the etheric level; as a result the healer's emotional state is very important. Etheric energy, which is channeled through the heart and projected as rays of energy, is experienced by the healer as intense feelings. These feelings serve as a feedback mechanism, which by their nature and intensity tell the healer the strength of the rays being projected to his patient. The more powerful the ray of energy projected through his heart chakra, the more love and compassion the healer feels for his patient. The more spiritual the healer's love, the higher the ray's rate of vibration. The ray of energy projected from the third eye is a projection of assertive energy from the intuitive, or unconscious mind. It is experienced by the healer as extreme clarity and will. The more energy the healer projects through his third eye, the more will power he will feel and the less distraction he will have during the healing session. When the heart and unconscious mind are working together and the remaining chakras are open and well balanced, the healer will be successful in projecting energy which will have a powerful healing effect on his patient. Edna St. Vincent Millay states:

> The heart can push the sea and land
> Farther away on either hand;
> The soul can split the sky in two,
> And let the face of God shine through.[47]

Projecting Rays of Energy

We start chakra healing in the same way we begin the
other forms of absentee healing, by entering the alpha/theta
level. Begin by finding a comfortable position, with your
back straight. Then close your eyes and begin the three
part Yogic breath. Continue breathing in this way for three
of four minutes, remembering not to separate inhalation
from exhalation. Continue until your breath becomes deep
and rhythmic. Then begin counting backwards from 5 to 1,
visualizing and repeating each number three times to yourself. When you reach the number 1, take a deep breath and
as you exhale, affirm to yourself, "I am now in the alpha
level, feeling better than I did before." Then take another
deep breath and count backwards from 10 to 1, going
deeper on each descending number. When you have reached
the number 1, mentally affirm, "Every time I come to this
level of mind I learn to use more of mind in more creative
ways". Next, take about five minutes to relax your physical body using one of the methods you learned earlier.
When you've finished relaxing your physical body, repeat
to yourself, "My body is completely relaxed; every time I
come to this level of mind I learn to go to deeper and
healthier levels." Then visualize yourself in your sanctuary
and remain there for the next five minutes. When you
return from your sanctuary, take a deep breath and on the
exhalation visualize your "visual screen" about six feet in
front of you, extending thirty degrees above your head.
Mentally repeat the name of your patient and he will
instantaneously appear on your screen. Once he is on your
screen, open your heart chakra and hold him on the
screen with love, compassion and empathy. You can do
this most easily by paying attention, breathing and putting the appropriate hand on your heart chakra.

Then, pay attention to your sixth chakra, the third
eye. By paying attention to it you will activate it, and
you will feel a tingling sensation as the chakra opens. You
may also feel a warm glowing sensation coming from it;
these are all indications the chakra is open and is trans-

mitting more prana through it.

Next, bring your breath to your third eye and let the prana, carried along with your breath, activate it further. Once you bring the breath to it, the sensations in the chakra will grow more intense. They will grow so strong that you will feel a ray of energy coming from it (this is one of the healing rays important in chakra healing). Focus your attention on the ray; it will be very defined like a laser. When you feel ready, project the ray of energy to your patient on the screen. Direct it to the part of his body which needs healing. Feel the ray of energy enter his body, going where it is most needed and feel your patient absorb the healing energy from the ray. Feel him take it in with gratitude and feel him relax as the energy has its healing effect on him. Remember that when you project energy to him, he is feeling its healing power on the etheric level, no matter where he is or what he is doing. (See plate)

Continue sending the healing ray from your third eye for three or four minutes. When you feel satisfied that it has had a positive effect, release the ray of energy from your third eye. Take a deep breath and go deeper. Then, direct your attention to your heart chakra and activate it mentally. You will begin feeling the energy from the fourth chakra grow in intensity once you apply mental attention to it. The fourth chakra will also feel warmer as the energy coming through it becomes stronger. Next, bring your breath to the heart and breathe from your heart without separation between inhalation and exhalation. The prana and air will activate it further. By now, you should feel strong feelings of compassion and love for your patient. It may be accompanied by an intense glowing or burning sensation (these are all manifestations of prana). Let the energy from your heart chakra become so strong that a ray of energy flows from it; it will feel more like a wave of energy, less distinct than the ray projected from your third eye, but full of love and power nonetheless. Feel the wave flow from your chakra to your patient and feel him absorb the energy with gratitude. See him smiling and in perfect,

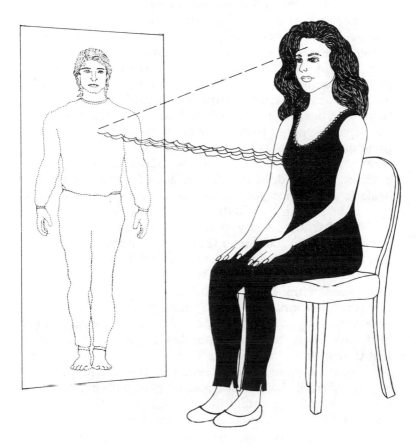

Plate 8: Projecting Healing Rays

radiant health as the energy has its healing effect. Continue projecting this ray for three or four minutes, or until you are satisfied.

Projecting the Rays Together
The rays of energy from the fourth and sixth chakras can be projected separately as we just did, but they have the greatest effect when they are combined and projected to a patient together. In the next part of chakra healing you will combine the ray of energy from your heart chakra with the ray of energy from your third eye, projecting them to your patient together. While you are projecting the wave of energy from your heart chakra, pay attention to your third eye as well. Dividing your attention in this way is simple to do and can be mastered with a little practice, but it does require an act of surrender on the healer's part. Once your attention is focused on the third eye, it will begin to vibrate. Then, bring the breath to it, and in a few moments you will feel the energy grow quite strong. Mentally focus it so that it joins the wave of energy from your heart chakra and feel both rays of energy being absorbed by the diseased tissue of your patient's body. Continue sending these rays of energy together for several minutes and empathize with your patient as the rays of energy have their healing effect on him. Continue sending both rays for three or four minutes, or until you feel satisfied they have had a healing effect.

You complete chakra healing by transferring the rays of energy from the diseased area of your patient's physical body to his etheric aura, filling his aura with the combined energy of the heart chakra and the third eye. Take a couple minutes to fill his aura with energy and vitality. His aura will expand and begin to glow as it fills with prana. After a minute or two, feel him absorb the energy through his skin and feel it recharging his entire body, even the cells themselves. Take two or three minutes to work on his aura and when you are finished, release the ray of energy from your heart chakra, and then let go of the ray of energy from your third eye. Release your patient and your visual screen. Take a deep breath and relax. In a few moments you will feel a wave of energy flow through your crown chakra. Allow it to recharge your entire subtle energy system. Take a couple minutes for recharging, continuing it until you feel your chakras glowing. When you are completely re-energized, mentally affirm, "Every time I act as a channel for healing, I am healed and I become a more effective channel for healing." Then return to normal consciousness by slowly counting from 1 to 5. When you reach the number 5, open your eyes. You will feel wide awake, perfectly relaxed and better than you did before.

Color Healing

There is a variation to this technique which you should begin using once you have mastered the one above. It is called color healing. It is identical to chakra healing, except that once you have combined the rays together, you project the rays of energy in color. This gives your patient the exact dosage or vibration of energy he needs, and will accelerate the healing process.

There are four major healing colors which I use in chakra healing: yellow, green, blue and violet. These colors have the most pronounced healing effect, although other colors can be beneficial. The secondary healing colors are orange, red, and pink. They should be used if your patient rejects the four major healing colors. The colors you project to your patient must always be clear and bright. Never send him dull, muddy or dirty colors. As you know from our study of the human aura, dirty, muddy colors are the colors of disease. Only bright colors are healing colors. There are no rules for determining which color will most benefit a particular patient. You must trust your intuition and treat each patient individually. Your intuition will tell you which color is the appropriate one in a given situation. Sometimes the appropriate color will appear spontaneously while you are projecting a single ray or both of them together. Sometimes your patient will show you which color he needs. If he does, you should follow your patient's instructions. If you start sending a particular color and you feel him resisting it, pushing it aside or just not absorbing it easily, then try another color and keep trying until you find the one he wants. The best time to begin using colors is after you have combined the energy from the third eye with the energy from the heart chakra. At first, wait to see if a healing color spontaneously appears; if it doesn't, begin experimenting with the four primary healing colors. Begin with yellow and go from there to green, then to blue and finally to violet. When you find the best color, stick with it for the duration of the healing.

Self-Healing with Color

Color can be very useful in self-healing as well. It can be used in two ways. If you have a local problem, one confined to a specific area of your body, you can use color in combination with visualization to treat it. To begin self-healing in this way, follow these instructions; find a comfortable position with your back straight and begin the three part Yogic breathing. Breathe Yogically until you feel very relaxed. Then slowly count backwards from 5 to 1. When you reach the number 1, mentally affirm, "I am now in the alpha level, feeling better than I did before." Then use a combination of techniques you learned earlier to put yourself firmly in the alpha/theta state.

When you are firmly in the alpha/theta state, begin paying attention to the afflicted area. Pay attention with your eyes open and try not to blink your eyes, but instead keep staring until they begin to unfocus spontaneously. This should only take a few moments (once your eyes are unfocused, blink them if necessary in order to avoid eye strain). When your eyes have unfocused, begin to visualize light surrounding the problem area. Begin with a clear white light and wait a few moments until the white light changes into one of the healing colors. This shouldn't take long. If at first colors don't appear, don't be discouraged, just begin experimenting with different colors that have healing properties. Continue experimenting with different colors until you find a color which is easily absorbed by your body. You should have no trouble visualizing, even with your eyes open, as long as they are unfocused and you remain in an alpha/theta state. Once you have the appropriate color and you feel it being absorbed, visualize the particular organ or tissue taking in the rays of energy and feel the cells being energized and healed as the energy is being absorbed by them.

Continue with this technique until you feel a sense of well-being flooding the problem area. You can use the breath to help you by feeling the diseased tissue absorbing the ray of energy on each inhalation, and on each exhalation feeling the healing energy radiating through the cells and recharging them. At first, take five minutes to do this form of self-healing. Then take two or three minutes to recharge yourself. When you have completed the recharging, mentally affirm, "I am in perfect health, perfect balance, and perfect harmony." Then return to the outer conscious level by slowly counting from 1 to 5. When you have reached the number 5, open your eyes. You will feel wide awake, perfectly relaxed and better than you did before. For the best results, practice this technique at least twice a day. Take about ten minutes to settle firmly into the alpha/theta level and spend at least five minutes doing self-healing.

Direct Self-Healing with Color

In another variation you can combine color healing, visualization and the magnetic energy which flows through your hands. Positive energy, which is assertive energy, flows through the right hand of all right handed people; it varies with left handed people, sometimes coming from the right hand and sometimes from the left hand, depending on how dominantly left handed a person is. For those of you who are left handed, start with your left hand and if the technique doesn't work, switch hands. To begin this variation, put the appropriate masculinely charged hand about two inches above the afflicted area, being careful to stay within your etheric aura. Close your eyes and begin the three part Yogic breath, breathing deeply without separation between inhalation and exhalation.

Using the appropriate appropriate method, put yourself into the alpha/theta level. When you are firmly in the alpha/theta level, pay attention to your masculine hand and activate it mentally until you feel your palm tingle and your hand gets warm. Next imagine a ray of energy flowing from your palm into the afflicted area. Use your breath to help you, the same way you did in the last variation. Begin by visualizing the ray as clear and wait until it changes color spontaneously. If it doesn't change after a few moments, experiment with the different healing colors until you find one that works best. Visualize the afflicted part or your body absorbing the ray of energy which comes through your hand. Feel it absorb the energy and feel the energy having its healing effect.

Continue with the technique for five minutes, or longer if you like. When you feel the technique has had a healing effect on the diseased tissue, remove your hand, take a deep breath and affirm to yourself, "I am being healed, and every day in every way I am getting healthier." Repeat the affirmation several times to yourself if you like. Take a few minutes to recharge and to enjoy the effects of the self-healing. When you are finished, complete your meditation with the affirmation, "I am in perfect health, I am in perfect balance, and I am in perfect harmony." Return to the outer conscious level by slowly counting from 1 to 5. When you reach 5, open your eyes. You will feel wide awake, perfectly relaxed and better than you did before.

Recharging your Aura with Colored Rays
The third variation in self-healing which I will explain is useful for problems that affect the entire body. It is especially beneficial in treating psychological and emotional problems. To start the variation, close your eyes and

begin breathing Yogically. Count backwards from 5 to 1, repeating and visualizing each number three times to yourself. When you have reached the number 1, affirm to yourself, "I am now deeply relaxed, feeling better than I did before." Continue with the Yogic breath and put yourself into the alpha/theta level using the techniques you learned earlier. Then begin the healing process by mentally repeating this affirmation, "I am now a channel for healing, and healing energy is flowing through me." Next, visualize your visual screen six feet in front of you, lift your gaze about thirty degrees and then repeat your own name to yourself, and you will see yourself appear on the screen. Hold yourself on the screen with love and compassion by opening your heart chakra. Pay attention to your third eye and breathe from it until you feel a ray of energy flowing from it filling your aura (the one on the screen) with energy. Pay attention to your heart chakra and feel a wave of energy flowing out from it. Feel it connect with the ray of energy from your third eye, and feel both rays together, filling your aura with healing energy. Wait a few moments to see if the rays change into one of the healing colors. If not, then experiment until you find the appropriate color for the healing. Continue sending the rays in color for the next five minutes. Imagine that your aura is getting bigger and brighter, until it looks like a large glowing egg surrounding you on the screen. Finally, imagine you are absorbing the energy and vitality from your aura through your skin and it is recharging and healing every cell in your body. Take as long as you like to complete this process. Finish it by seeing yourself on the screen as perfectly happy and healthy, smiling radiantly. Complete the visualization by affirming to yourself, "I am in perfect health; I am in perfect balance; I am in perfect harmony." Return to the outer conscious level by slowly counting from 1 to 5. When you open your eyes you will feel wide awake, perfectly relaxed and better than you did before.

Empathy and Self-Healing

As you already know, in all forms of healing it is important to empathize with your patient. This is especially true in self-healing. Empathy is a form of communion with another being. It can only happen when a person feels so much for another that he experiences life as the other person does, by feeling his feelings and thinking his thoughts. In self-healing empathy is very important, but it can only be achieved if you can detach yourself from your own suffering; only in that way can you, the healer, empathize with the patient. Detachment from your own suffering is essential in self-healing, because only then can the I AM emerge, (the I AM is free from disease on every level) and empathize with the "you" who needs healing. When you learn detachment, the I AM which channels healing energy from God transmutes your disease and suffering into perfect health and joy. Cultivate detachment and let the power of the All pour into you; by doing so you will be healing yourself and you will be on your way to perfect health, harmony and balance. We read in the *Vedas*:

> God being one, and
> concealed in the depth of every being,
> is the soul of all.
> He is the ruler and ordainer of all actions;
> He is the residence of all
> and the witness of all;
> He is the cause of
> all consciousness, (yet)
> He is without title
> and without any attribute.
> He is the secondless one,
> and also the soul,
> of every individual existence
> (both of matter and life).
> He is the one who changes
> one seed into various growths.
> Those who are able to perceive him
> as one existing in the depth
> of their own intellect,

they and they alone become
the receivers of eternal happiness,
none other (can become as such).
He is without any part
and without any action;
He is without any wrong
and is without any attachment;
He is the bridge to freedom,
and He is the peaceful;
like the fire without fuel,
He is without any title and
He is radiant and effulgent.
Trying to end sorrow
Without knowing him,
is like trying to encircle
the sky with leather.
(That means it is impossible
to end sorrow without knowing him).[48]

CHAPTER TWELVE

THE COMPLETE ABSENTEE HEALING

In this chapter you will be using the absentee healing techniques you have learned in earlier chapters to perform a complete absentee healing combining affirmation, visualization, psychic diagnosis, chakra healing and color healing.

Going to the Alpha/Theta Level

To begin a complete absentee healing, find a comfortable position, either sitting with your back straight or lying down. Close your eyes and begin breathing Yogically. Continue the Yogic breathing for three or four minutes and feel the internal chatter (which indicates beta level activity) quiet down. When you feel the sense of well-being associated with the alpha/theta state, begin counting backwards from 5 to 1. On each descending number, repeat and visualize the number three times to yourself. When you reach the number 1 mentally affirm, "I am now deeply relaxed, feeling better than I did before."

Continue with the Yogic breath and when you are ready, count backwards from 10 to 1, exhaling as you mentally say 10 . . . take another deep breath, and while exhaling, mentally repeat the number 9 . . . another deep breath, and while exhaling, mentally say 8 . . . continuing in this manner until you reach the number 1. By the time you reach the number 1, you will be feeling very light and clear. Pay attention to the subtle changes which you feel in your physical, emotional and mental body. When you reach the number 1, mentally affirm, "Every time I come to this level of mind, I learn to use more of my mind in more creative ways."

Relaxing the Physical Body

To relax your physical body completely, you can use the ancient Yogic practice you learned earlier to release the tension stored within your voluntary muscles. By releasing all tension you will ensure the free passage of prana through your subtle energy system. When you are ready, exhale completely and pay attention to your feet. Then inhale and tighten the muscles of your feet as much as possible. Hold your breath for three seconds. After three seconds, release your breath and allow the muscles of your feet to relax. Inhale deeply again and repeat the procedure, this time with the ankles and calves. Repeat the procedure with the following parts of your body: the thighs, the buttocks and pelvis, the middle and upper abdomen, the chest and shoulders, the neck, the hands, the arms; then squeeze the muscles of your face and hold for three seconds. After three seconds, release and exhale. Next, open your mouth, stick out your tongue and stretch the muscles of your face as much as possible; hold your breath for three seconds, then release the muscles of your face and exhale.

To complete the relaxation, contract your entire body all at once (this time, squeezing the muscles of your face), keeping them tight while holding your breath. After three seconds, expel the air forcibly and release all the muscles of your body at once.

Your Sanctuary

About ten minutes will have elapsed by this time, and you should be firmly in the alpha/theta level. Continue by mentally affirming, "I am in the alpha level. Every time I come to this level of mind, it makes it easier for me to go to deeper and healthier levels." Let your mind drift to your sanctuary, your perfect place of relaxation. Enjoy your sanctuary for five minutes.

The Visual Screen

When you return from your sanctuary, mentally affirm, "I am a channel for healing, and healing energy is flowing through me." Visualize your visual screen six feet in front of you, rising thirty degrees above your head. Look upward thirty degrees, and mentally repeat the name of your patient. He will instantaneously appear on your screen. Hold your patient on the screen by paying attention to your heart chakra, breathing from it and placing your hand on it.

Psychic Diagnosis

Once your patient is firmly on the screen, begin scanning his body for medical problems. Let your intuition be your guide and go anywhere it takes you. You will be attracted to areas where there is disease. If your attention is drawn to a particular part of the body, first examine the aura above the area and check for problems in its color, texture and shape. If there is a problem with the aura, continue your investigation by projecting your consciousness below it into the diseased organ or tissue. Examine the diseased tissue for abnormalities. Remember, empathy is important if you want to see your patient's problem in its fullness. Complete your diagnosis with a complete scan of your patient's aura and physical body. Watch for any other abnormalities and if you find any, repeat the procedure above.

Chakra Healing

When you complete your diagnosis, take several deep breaths and feel yourself going deeper. Begin mentally talking to your patient, reassuring him until he becomes completely relaxed and receptive to the healing energy you project. Then pay attention to your third eye and activate it mentally. When you feel the chakra tingle, glow and get warm, bring your breath to it and breathe from it. This will activate it even further. The sensations in the sixth chakra will grow so strong that a ray of energy will emerge.

When this happens, direct the ray of energy to the diseased area of your patient's body. Feel your patient absorb the energy, taking it in with gratitude. Then bring your attention to your heart chakra and mentally activate it. When you feel the chakra tingle and begin to glow, start breathing from it and let your mind and breath activate it further. The energy in the chakra will grow in strength until you feel a wave of energy emerge from it. When this happens, direct the wave of energy to the diseased area of your patient's body. Feel the combined energy from both chakras being absorbed by your patient. Feel him taking in the energy with gratitude.

Color Healing

Once you have combined the rays of energy, wait for them to spontaneously change from clear to one of the healing colors. If they don't change in a few moments, then experiment with one of the primary healing colors: yellow, green, blue or violet. If your patient doesn't absorb one of these colors easily, try one of the secondary healing colors: orange, pink or red. Make sure the color you project is clear and bright. When you find the right color, continue with chakra and color healing for three or four minutes. When you feel satisfied the rays have had a healing effect, release the ray of energy from your third eye. Then release the ray of energy from your heart chakra.

Mental Healing

Keep the image of your patient on the screen for another few moments with the love and compassion which is flowing through your heart. Take a deep breath and for the next few moments feel yourself going deeper. Bring your attention and your breath to your third chakra, the solar plexus. Your attention and breath will activate it and you will feel a vibration going through the chakra. The vibration will increase until you feel the chakra getting warm and beginning to tingle. As the intensity grows stronger, visualize a cord emerging from the chakra connecting you with your patient. Feel the cord stretching from your solar plexus to his solar plexus. Feel yourself being pulled into your patient and visualize the cord between you getting shorter as you get closer to each other. Let go completely and allow yourself to be drawn into your patient's physical body. Then mentally affirm, "I am standing by the (insert name of diseased tissue) ready to perform healing." Instantaneously you will be standing beside the diseased tissue. Imagine that you have a set of tools with you that you can use for healing your patient. Take about five minutes to heal the diseased area with your tools. When you have finished and you visualize the tissue in a state of perfect health, mentally put your hands opposite each other on the once diseased tissue and pay attention to your masculinely charged hand. Once you activate the hand mentally, you will feel it get hot and begin to vibrate. When this happens, feel a ray of energy flowing from your masculinely charged hand and feel the energy being absorbed by the once diseased tissue. Take a couple minutes and mentally explain to your patient that this extra healing energy will protect the area and will keep it in good health.

Recharging your Patient's Aura

When you are satisfied with your work and the diseased area has returned to a state of perfect health, visualize yourself standing outside your patient's body about six feet in front of your visual screen. Take a deep breath and feel yourself going deeper. Bring your attention and your breath to your third eye and activate it until you feel a ray of energy emerge. Feel the ray of energy flowing from your chakra into your patient's aura and then follow the same procedure with your heart chakra until you feel energy emerge from it and you feel it connect with the energy coming from your third eye. Feel both rays pouring energy into your patient's aura, recharging it and revitalizing it. Allow the rays of energy to change into the most effecive healing color and watch your patient's aura glow and expand as the healing energy pours into it. When his aura is saturated with energy, feel him absorb the energy through his skin, and feel the energy radiating through the body, healing and re-energizing every cell. Project energy into the aura in this way for two or three minutes or until you feel satisfied. When you are finished, release the ray of energy from your third eye, and release the ray of energy from your heart chakra. Then visualize your patient surrounded by radiant light; smiling, happy, full of vitality and in perfect health.

Recharging Yourself

When you are done, release your patient and release your visual screen. Take a deep breath and mentally affirm, "Every time I act as a channel for healing, not only is my patient healed, but I am healed as well." Take the next two or three minutes to recharge your subtle energy system. You will know your subtle energy system is completely recharged when you feel your chakras glowing. In the beginning you may only feel a glowing sensation in your crown chakra and third eye, but as you become more sensitive to the different frequencies of energy in your body, you will feel the other chakras glowing as well. When you are satisfied you are completely recharged, mentally affirm, "Every time I send healing to another person I become a more powerful channel for healing." Then slowly count from 1 to 5. When you reach the number 5, open your eyes. You will feel wide awake, perfectly relaxed and better than you did before.

CHAPTER THIRTEEN

QUESTIONS ABOUT ABSENTEE HEALING

Over the years I have been asked many questions about absentee healing. I would like to answer some of the most common ones for you. My answers to these questions are based on my own experience, not on any rigid doctrine or theology. They are subjective and in the end you must let your own intuition and conscience guide you.

Multiple Healings

Question one: is it a good idea to work on more than one person during a healing meditation? The answer to this depends on the healer, the amount of time he has available for absentee healing and his level of vitality. Vitality depends on several things; the healer's ability to surrender to the healing force, his ability to store prana, and of course his state of mental, emotional and physical health. The only rule to follow is, "never strain". If you feel that healing has become an effort, if afterwards you are exhausted, or if at the end of the day you feel a lack of vitality, then you have done too many healings that day and should cut down. You will find that after you are healing for just a short time, your capacity will increase and you will be able to work with more patients for longer periods of time.

Resistent Patients

Question two: should a healer work on people without their permission or who don't want to be healed?

I have always worked on anyone I intuitively felt would
benefit from spiritual healing. This means I don't work on
everyone who comes to me. I can tell those people who
won't benefit from spiritual healing and I don't work on
them. I do work on people who haven't asked me to work
on them, or who are resistant. My decisions have always
been based on my intuition and then scrutinized by my
conscience. When I get the OK from both, I work on someone and I will not be put off by anyone or anything. Intuition and conscience are both manifestations of the inner
self, the I AM, which is linked directly to God.

The Apostle Paul, himself a great channel for healing,
tells us, "For we are his workmanship, created in Christ
Jesus unto good works, which God hath before ordained
that we should walk in them.[49] I believe as Paul did that
God, the All, has set before us works to do. These works
can only be recognized when we are aware of them. Awareness of these works can only come if we pay attention, and
follow our intuition. God does the healing, knows who will
be healed and when they will be healed. Only by paying
attention will you know which patients He has chosen for
you. If you feel intuitively you should work with someone,
there is a great likelihood your work will benefit him. Even
if he consciously doesn't want healing, send healing energy
anyway. He may not consciously want it, but unconsciously
he may be desperately crying out for it.

The Length of a Healing Session

Question three: how long should an absentee healing
session last? There is no standard length of time for an
absentee healing. I combine absentee healing with meditation, and the entire process takes about forty minutes. It
might differ with you and that's fine. In a forty minute
meditation I take about fifteen minutes for the actual
healing. This is an average. Sometimes I take more time,
and sometimes less depending upon how I feel. In "laying
on of hands" I usually spend about thirty minutes doing
the actual healing. But I have worked for far less time

when conducting a workshop or doing things in public.
You must remember, time itself is not the most important factor in healing. I've seen people healed instantaneously after being touched for only a few seconds.

How Long Before the Patient is Healed

Question four: how long does it take for a complete
physical healing? The healer never knows for sure how
long a physical healing will take. The Hermetic philosophy
teaches us that healing is a process of transmutation; energy
from the higher planes is transmuted for the purpose of
healing, but in many cases this takes time. It may also take
time for the patient's physical body to transmute healing
energy and use it for healing physical disease. Also, healing the mind and the emotions is often a prerequisite for
physical healing. Although we aim for immediate results,
in many cases it is unrealistic to expect an immediate
physical healing when a patient's mental body and etheric
(emotional) body are still diseased. Many healers work
over long periods of time with patients before they see the
desired results. In 1981 I had such an experience. I was
asked to work on a man who suffered from a serious eye
disorder; because of it he had lost his peripheral vision.
He was left with tunnel vision only. To compound matters,
the gentleman suffered from hemmorhages in both eyes
which further distorted his vision. Neither of his conditions
could be treated by traditional medical means. He was 82
years old when I met him, and with the exception of his
eyes he was in excellent health. Before meeting me he had
no interest in or knowledge about spiritual healing. He was
not a religious man, and I was the first healer he had ever
met. We began working together twice a week, and I also
included him in my daily healing meditations. At first,
because of his anxiety, he had difficulty taking in the full
amount of energy I was channeling to him. On most occa-
sions I had to push through blockages before the healing
energy would get through. Projecting color was particularly
difficult at first, and so was chakra healing. His lack of

receptivity also made visualization difficult. My intuition told me to continue working with him, and I did, using whichever techniques proved most effective. After the first month, things slowly began to change. The blockages began to fall away, and little by little my visualizations became more vivid and protracted. Soon I felt a rapport being established between us. By the fifth week he began to accept some color, and the connection between us grew more solid, until I could feel him in his "fullness". After six weeks of work neither of us could see any tangible improvement in his physical condition. He was not discouraged by the initial lack of results, and even without seeing progress he was determined to carry on. Six weeks into treatment he went to see his eye doctor for his regular bi-annual check up and he was told, to his amazement, that his vision had improved. He couldn't see the improvement at that point, but he was greatly encouraged and so was I. We continued to work together with a renewed enthusiasm, and within one week he began to experience a change in his vision. First the improvement lasted only a few hours, but by the end of the seventh week of treatment, the improvement became more protracted and the distortion began to disappear. He went back to his doctor at the end of the eighth week and he was told there was a remarkable change in his vision. Not only had the distortion stopped, but so had the hemmorhages. We continued to work and the tunnel vision began to improve. For the first time in months he began to read again, first with a magnifying glass, but a short time later without one. He began to play cards again and to watch television, neither of which he could do before. Between the sixth and tenth week of treatment, his doctor estimated he had regained 80% of his sight.

We are told the Earl of Sandwich had the healing touch, and that he worked for extended periods of time with his patients. Archibald Holms in his book, *The Facts of Psychic Science* tells us that in 1908 the Earl discovered he had healing ability. "Lord Sandwich did not make cures

of the miraculous type, he was however remarkably successful in banishing pain; and although the disease might
not be cured, the pain in many cases did not recur. Lord
Sandwich made many cures among the poor and suffering;
his treatment was often protracted, and so self-sacrificing
was he that sometimes he saw the poor sufferer every day
for a year or more."[50]

The Best Times for Healing

Question five: when is the best time to perform healing? There isn't one answer which can be applied to all
conditions and all circumstances. Each of us has a different
life style that must be taken into consideration. Of course
I recommend you work when you are relaxed, when you
have nothing pressing on your mind. It is not a good idea
to work when you are rushed or sleepy. I usually recommend to my students that they perform absentee healing
in the early evening after they've completed their day's
work. If your schedule permits, you can work in the morning also. Remember that the more time you work on a
patient the better. The Bible seconds this by telling us,
"The effective fervent prayer of a righteous man availeth
much."[51] Finally, I tell students that although they perform
healing meditations twice a day, it doesn't mean they can't
do absentee healing while they are engaged in other activities. You might be focusing your conscious mind on one
thing, but you can still send healing to someone who needs
it, with your unconscious mind. You can do this any time
you want. While walking down the street you may see
someone in pain; send him healing. At work someone may
be suffering; send him healing as well. It doesn't matter
what activities you're engaged in. It is possible to be consciously active and still project healing energy. Simply
begin by going into the alpha/theta state, which becomes
easy once you practice healing regularly. The fastest way
is to affirm you are in the alpha/theta state and healing
energy is coming through you. Then pay attention to your
fourth and sixth chakras, and feel healing rays flowing

to your patient. Once rapport is established, go right into affirmation and visualization. I assure you that with a little practice, you will be able to perform healing anytime and anywhere.

CHAPTER FOURTEEN

LAYING ON OF HANDS

Everywhere you turn, history gives evidence of spiritual healing through the "laying on of hands". It is often used in combination with other techniques, such as anointing with oils, magnetizing cloth, cotton, water, and other natural substances. Sometimes direct contact is made with saliva and clay as described in the New Testament, "As Jesus passed by, he saw a man who was blind from his birth . . . he spat on the ground, and made clay of the spittle, and anointed the eyes of the blind man with clay and said unto him, Go, wash in the pool of Siloam . . . he went his way, therefore, and washed, and came seeing."[52]

Sometimes the healing is done directly when the healer touches the patient's physical body. Sometimes in laying on of hands the healer works only on the patient's etheric aura without making physical contact. Usually, it is the healer who does the touching, but this is not always the case. The patient can initiate the healing by touching the healer, or simply by coming within the healer's auric field. This remarkable healing from the New Testament will illustrate:

> And a certain woman, which had an issue of blood twelve years, and had suffered many things of many physicians, and had spent all that she had, and was nothing bettered, but rather grew worse, when she had heard of Jesus, came in the crowd behind, and touched his garment.

141

For she said, if I may touch but his clothes, I shall
be whole. And straightway the fountain of her
blood was dried up, and she felt in her body that
she was healed of that plague. And Jesus ... turned
him about in the crowd, and said, Daughter, thy
faith hath made thee whole; go in peace and be
whole of the plague.[53]

History of Laying On of Hands

"Laying on of hands" is the preferred method of the
vast majority of healers. It has been called the "king's
touch" and it was known as that in medieval France and
England. We are told the Roman Emperors Vespasian and
Hadrian had such a gift. So did the Norwegian King Olaf,
who in his time was considered a saint. St. Patrick was able
to heal the sick through laying on of hands. It is reported
he healed the blind in Ireland by placing his hands on their
eyes. The early Greeks were aware a sick person could be
healed through the laying on of hands. Hippocrates tells
us, "It is believed by many experienced doctors that the
heat which oozes out of the hand, on being applied to the
sick, is highly salutary and assuaging."[54]

In ancient Egypt laying on of hands was practiced
from the earliest times, being the domain of the temple
priests. It was extensively practiced in the temples of Isis,
Osiris and Serapis. Scholars and Egyptologists have found
representations of direct healing on sarcophagi, jewelry
and on wall paintings. It was handed down to them by the
early Hermeticists who practiced it as part of the ancient
mystery cults. Even to this day we can see laying on of
hands as part of the healing practices of the Rosicrucians
and Masons, both of whom trace their lineage back to
ancient Egypt. Its universality and antiquity is undisputed.
Evidence of its practice has been traced back more than
fifteen thousand years, where evidence of it has been discovered in Neolithic cave paintings in the Pyrenees. Healing by direct contact, or what we call laying on of hands,
appears to be a universal human practice. It has never been

confined to any sect or region, nor has any religious group had a monopoly on it. It has been practiced in India, China, ancient Israel, Chaldea, as well as in the West, even before the time of Christ. It flourished throughout the Middle Ages inside and outside the orthodox church, and has been practiced by shamans and brujos throughout the Third World to the present day. It is only in the West, with the beginning of the Industrial Revolution and the Age of Reason, that the laying on of hands fell into disrepute. Even in the West, small groups like the Theosophists and Pentecostals have kept the tradition alive. Healings have continued unabated in these and other sects, sometimes spilling over into the general population.

Who Can Do Laying On of Hands

Anyone with a sincere desire and a real interest can use his mind and hands for healing. He doesn't have to join any organization or become involved in any cult or espouse any particular doctrine. The only prerequisite for practicing laying on of hands is a sincere concern and empathy for the health and happiness of others. Knowledge is important, but experience is the best teacher. Make an honest appraisal of your own physical and mental health, and as long as you don't think either one will get in the way, you can begin helping others by practicing direct healing. In one of his trance readings, Edgar Cayce was asked by a woman participating in a healing group, "Please clarify our minds as to the methods and ways for us to proceed in our seeking to help others." His answer was lengthy, but this excerpt gives us the essence of his reply, ". . . use what thou has in hand, day by day. Knowledge and understanding comes along with application, and with self's experience in doing what is known to be in accord with His will."[55]

Never Be Discouraged

Many people who suffer from physical disease are discouraged from working with others. I feel this is unfortunate. This excerpt from the *Life of St. Augustine* will illustrate why. Possidius, his biographer, relates that just before Augustine's death while he was suffering his last illness, "A certain man came with a sick relative and asked him to lay his hand upon him that he might be cured. Augustine replies that, if he had any such power, he certainly would have first applied it to himself. Thereupon, his visitor replied that he had a vision and in his sleep heard these words, 'Go to Bishop Augustine that he may lay his hand upon him and he will be healed.' When Augustine learned this, he did not delay doing it, and immediately the Lord caused the sick man to depart from him healed."[56]

Attitude and Environment

I mentioned earlier that faith is an essential ingredient in healing, and I don't mean just the faith of the healer. It is the faith of the patient, all things being equal, which guarantees success in healing. Everything the healer does must be done with this fact in mind. In direct healing, the healer comes into personal contact with his patient. As a result, he must do only those things which nurture his patient's trust in him, and in the process of spiritual healing.

The healer must have confidence in himself and must inspire confidence in his patients. Arrogance, haughtiness and egotism have no place in healing. Remember, healing comes from God, and you are His instrument with a sacred function to perform.

When you meet your patient for the first time, fill him with confidence and assure him he can be healed. Through affirmations, plant in him the *idée fixe* he will recover. In place of hopelessness, inspire him to work along with you with courage and enthusiasm. Encourage him to persevere even though at first there may be no evidence of improvement. I have found in a majority of cases that perceptible improvement often takes a little while. Remember your patient has come to you for help and he is susceptible to suggestion; nurture his initial hope until he becomes convinced beyond doubt he will be healed.

If nourished, the conviction will blossom into faith, and as we know, with faith all things are possible.

Direct healing should be practiced in a quiet, serene environment where there are no disruptions. The healer should put aside sufficient time before and after the healing to talk to his patient and explain the techniques he will be using. Even more important, the healer should listen to his patient. The healer should allow his patient to unburden himself before the healing. It is highly unlikely that anyone suffering physically would be free from emotional and psychological pain; the healer must remember there is a direct connection between good health and his patient's emotional and mental state. The healer is responsible for the total person when he performs a healing, not just his patient's physical body. Therefore, developing a wholistic approach is essential. When the patient is sufficiently relaxed, the healer ought to explain in a simple manner the techniques he will be using and how they will affect his patient; nothing should be left out.

Preparing the Patient

On my patient's first visit I ask him if he knows anything about spiritual healing. About twenty per cent have some knowledge of spiritual healing, homeopathy or wholistic medicine. However, for the majority of people, spiritual healing is an entirely new area. Most people, having been brought up in the rational, intellectual environment of America and Western Europe are usually trained from childhood to believe that only what they see is real. Their concept of disease and their responsibility for it is often at odds with the concepts of metaphysics and spiritual healing. As gently as possible, I explain what spiritual healing is without being controversial, showing the person as clearly as possible that my system is not at odds with modern medicine, but is an essential part of it. I explain he can participate in his own healing, and he no longer has to be victimized by his condition, no matter how or when it originated.

I tell him there are three different techniques I will be using in laying on of hands: vibrational healing, polarization, and empathetic healing. I explain that these techniques have variations which include different hand movements. After we have talked and I have explained the theory behind healing and what he should expect during the healing session, I have him lie down. I give him a few moments to get comfortable, and then ask him to close his eyes and relax. After a few moments, I ask him to begin breathing deeply and I guide him into the three part Yogic breath. Breathing correctly helps him to relax and it helps set the right mood for healing. Once my patient is breathing deeply and he is relaxed, I tell him what feelings and sensations he can expect when the healing begins. I tell him which parts of the body I will be touching, etc. I explain that healing energy is experienced in different ways; it is often experienced as intense heat coming from the healer's hands. But healing energy isn't always experienced as heat. Sometimes patients feel the energy as "cold rays" coming from the healer's hands. It can also be experienced as a tingle or vibration in the area the healer is touching. Sometimes the tingling sensations run through the extremities. The patient sometimes feels very light headed, dizzy, or becomes momentarily disoriented. In most cases, the sensations experienced during laying on of hands will differ from the normal physical condition. In some of my cases, however,where there was a noticeable improvement or even complete healing, the patient felt nothing unusual except a deep sense of relaxation.

Preparing Yourself for Direct Healing
Before I make direct contact with my patient, I make sure I am in the right state to be an effective channel. I ensure this by breathing yogically, and mentally repeating affirmations which bring me into a deep alpha level. Once I am in the alpha state, I mentally affirm, "I am a channel for healing, and healing energy is coming through me." I sometimes repeat this affirmation several times. Then I

place my hands on the patient's temples. I always begin laying on of hands with the head, and end with the head.

I spend about five minutes working directly on my patient's head, using vibrational healing. Then I move to the diseased part of my patient's body and work there for about fifteen minutes using vibrational, polarity and empathetic healing; often combining these techniques with hand movements and absentee healing techniques. Then I return to my patient's head and spend five minutes using a combination of healing techniques to complete the session. After I have entered the alpha state and I have put my hands on my patient's head, I begin healing through vibration. It is always the first technique I use in laying on of hands.

The Importance of Vibration

The third Hermetic axiom provides us with the metaphysical basis for vibrational healing. It tell us that, "Nothing rests; everything moves; everything vibrates."[57] Many healers are consciously aware of the healing vibration running through their etheric body. I call it the central pranic vibration. I experience it whenever I am functioning in the alpha/theta state. It becomes very pronounced when I do direct healing.

Vibration is important for us in healing because the strength of the central pranic vibration is directly related to the amount of prana flowing through a healer's subtle energy system, and the strength of the vibration determines the amount of energy which the healer has available for direct healing. I have observed that students engaged in direct healing via vibration have clearer, brighter, and larger etheric auras than before they began vibrational healing. Also, there is a shift in color in their aura from reds and yellows to greens and blues. Interestingly, students have told me that while they are doing vibrational healing, they feel light headed and their chakras began glowing; some reported their aura felt bigger or got warmer. Others said they felt they were on fire, or their head grew larger and larger once they achieved the vibrational state.

The vibrational state with its increased energy level facilitates the healer's ability to visualize. The healer's mind is cleared of useless chatter once the vibration is achieved so he can work without distraction. Moreover, once the healer has achieved the state of vibration, it is easier for him to work from the heart chakra, because he will find it easier to "think from the heart". The Bible tells us it is from the heart that "the love of God is shed abroad,"⁵⁸ and it is through the heart the healing force is most powerfully manifested. Thinking from the heart should not be confused with feelings which come from the heart. Feelings will be associated with the thoughts from the heart, but they are not actual thinking, which is the result of transmuting the desire of the heart into love. Thinking from the heart is motivated by love and compassion, and the sincere desire to see another person healthy and happy. It can only be achieved when the healer has developed his mental capacities to a sufficiently high state. Then he will radiate his healing charisma continually like "rivers of living water."⁵⁹

Of the three kinds of direct healing, vibrational healing has the most immediate effect on the patient. As soon as the healer achieves the vibrational state, the patient will feel a surge of energy, often accompanied by tingling sensations in his body. He will also experience an immediate improvement in his sense of well-being.

Achieving the Vibrational State

You can quickly achieve the vibrational state and begin vibrational healing by practicing the following breathing exercises. The technique is similar to the Yogic breath. Once you have begun laying on of hands by placing your hands on your patient's temples, begin breathing deeply without separation between inhalation and exhalation. Then pay attention to the rhythms of your body and allow your bodily rhythms to direct the rhythm of your breathing. This should take one or two minutes. Thinking from the heart will magnify the unconscious rhythms of your physical body and the subtle energy system, and will bring them into consciousness. Allow these internal rhythms to direct your breathing, and then bring your attention to your hands. Your breath should be slightly forced, and you should continue breathing without separation between inhalation and exhalation until you feel your hands vibrate and get hot.

After a short time, which could be from thirty seconds to five minutes, depending on how adept you are at this technique, you should begin to feel a deep, almost overwhelming compassion for your patient. Your hands will be vibrating so strongly that even without special breathing they will continue to vibrate. Once the vibration becomes self-sustaining, begin to breathe normally and allow your conscious mind to wander, while you keep your attention on your hands. The vibration will begin to lessen in your hands after a minute or two, but it will trigger a deeper, more important vibration (the central pranic vibration) which you will notice first in your chest cavity or at least somewhere in the central part of your body. It will be more subtle than the vibration in your hands.

If you pay attention, you will feel the central pranic vibration increase in strength, and you will feel it radiate through your entire body. Unlike the initial vibration which wears off as soon as your breathing returns to normal, the central pranic vibration will continue for as long as you pay attention to it. It is the second vibration which the healer wants to activate during each session of vibrational healing. This vibration is directly related to thinking from the heart, and although the initial vibration has curative effects in itself, its main function is to initiate the second vibration.

Don't concentrate on the second vibration. If you do, you will disrupt it. Keep thinking from the heart. The vibration is self-sustaining. After awhile, the central pranic vibration will move into your hands, and they will begin to vibrate again. When this happens, keep your hands on your

patient's head for just a minute or two longer. Then move
your hands from your patient's head to the afflicted area.
Don't move abruptly. Continue thinking from the heart
even while you are changing position. Once you've changed
position, place your hands on either side of the problem
area (remember to keep them apart) and continue healing
with this technique for three or four mintues, letting your
heart guide you, and allowing the vibration to flow through
your subtle energy system into your patient. Other healing
techniques will spontaneously appear during vibrational
healing. They will not interfere with the vibration, and I
encourage you to use mental healing, chakra healing and
color healing along with vibrational healing, especially
when you are working on the diseased area of your patient's
body. If these techniques don't appear spontaneously, program for them. Remember that programming is never done
with any effort, so there should be no problem with maintaining the central pranic vibration during the programming.
The unconscious mind will still apply its undivided attention to healing, maintaining the loving connection with the
patient as you think from the heart, while the conscious
mind, which has been given free rein to drift, is brought
back into service. At this point you can return to your
patient's head and work on his head for another four or
five minutes. Then you can return to normal consciousness
using the techniques you learned in absentee healing, or
you can continue working on the diseased area using the
stroking technique described next, or one of the other
direct healing techniques you will learn in the next two
chapters.

Vibration and Stroking

Vibrational healing is always done by making direct
contact with your patient's body. However, there is a variation which you can use while working in your patient's
etheric aura. It consists of stroking movements which you
make with your hands. I have found the most effective
time for using stroking is right after the initial vibration

has dissipated and after you have finished working on the diseased area.

Stroking can be done in a number of ways, but no matter which way the hands are used, it is essential for you to keep thinking from the heart and to focus the energy coming from your hands to the appropriate area of your patient's body. Stroking is initiated by lifting your hands from your patient's body, keeping them within the etheric aura about two or three inches above the physical body. Then with your hands apart and fingers spread, make a long fluid pass along the entire length of your patient's body from head to foot. You'll probably have to stand up to do this. Hold your breath while you are making the pass, inhaling just as you begin, and exhaling when you've completed the pass at your patient's feet.

You should make seven passes when you use this technique, and when you've completed each pass you should shake your hands away from your patient in order to remove any negativity which you might have picked up as you made the pass through his aura. When you've completed the seven passes, return to your original position at the head of your patient.

Recharging your Patient's Aura

When you have finished the seven passes, return to his head and place your hands on his temples again with the hands opposite each other. Take a couple of minutes to mentally fill your patient's aura with rays of energy from your heart chakra and third eye. Continue with the combined use of chakra healing and vibrational healing until your patient's aura is bursting with energy and vitality. Feel him absorb the energy through his skin and feel it recharging every cell in his body. Feel him take it in with gratitude. Visualize him happy, healthy and smiling radiantly. When you've finished the session of direct healing, remove your hands from your patient's head and tell your patient to remain where he is with his eyes closed. Explain it is part of the healing process, and by remaining quiet and relaxed he will absorb the healing energy more easily. While the patient remains quiet you should take a few moments to recharge your chakras the same way you did in absentee healing. Mentally affirm, "Every time I perform direct healing, not only is my patient healed, but I am healed as well." Return to normal consciousness by counting slowly from 1 to 5. When you reach the number 5, open your eyes and you will feel wide awake, perfectly relaxed and better than you did before.

Cleansing

Once your chakras are fully charged, you should do this simple cleansing to remove any residual negativity which you might have picked up while doing laying on of hands. It is done by simply immersing your hands in cold running water three times. After each immersion, briskly shake the water from your hands and mentally affirm, "Negativity has no effect on me on any level." At the end of the third immersion your hands should feel a little tingly and there should be a light, pleasant feeling in them. There should be no trace of negativity in your hands, or anywhere else in your body once the cleansing is complete.

After the Healing Is Over

After the cleansing, return to your patient and have him sit up. Give him some time to tell you what he experienced. Remember that any unusual experience indicates healing energy has affected him. Be encouraging if he tells you he felt something unusual during the healing. If he is not spontaneously healed, explain that healing is a progression. He must be patient and wait for the energy to be transmuted from his subtle energy system to his physical body. Explain that it may take a little while for the transmutation to be completed.

The Healer's Reaction

I am often asked how the healer should feel after a direct healing session. The answer is fairly simple. If the healer remains detached by keeping his ego out of the way, he will feel invigorated and relaxed afterwards. I feel the residual effects of the healing for hours. By acting as a channel for healing energy, the healer benefits from the energy as it flows through his subtle energy system. If the healer does several healings in a row, however, he might feel a mild dissipation which is caused by an excess expenditure of personal vitality. With every healing, there is a small expenditure of the healer's prana which must be differentiated from the Divine healing energy (prana) which is channeled through the healer during healing. This loss is inconsequential when only one or two healings are done. When a healer does several healings in one day, there will sometimes be a drain of personal prana. This drain will affect his nervous system and it will be experienced as an unusual form of exhaustion, sometimes making the healer feel lethargic or sleepy. This situation in itself is not dangerous if the healer allows himself time to naturally recharge. If the healer organizes his schedule with this in mind, allowing himself ample time to rest, play and sleep, by the next day he should be completely recharged and full of vitality.

The most enjoyable way I know to recharge yourself if you become drained is to walk barefoot either on the beach or in a field. A leisurely ten minute walk will have amazing effects. All natural environments have a restorative quality, as do small children and animals. Eating wholesome foods and natural vegetables will provide you with prana; so will clear, natural water. Use whatever combination of these which is suitable if you become exhausted and be sure to breathe deeply. In a short time you will be ready to perform direct healing again.

CHAPTER FIFTEEN

POLARIZATION

The second part of direct healing I call polarization. It can be understood in terms of the seventh Hermetic axiom which states, "Gender is in everything; everything has its masculine and femine principles; gender manifests on all planes."[60]

As we know, the masculine principle is assertive, while the feminine is receptive. For the healer, this duality has important implications. I discovered its importance early in my work when I found that if I prayed for an extended period of time with devotion, opening my heart and emoting deep feelings of love and empathy, my body became extremely energized and I would feel waves of energy flowing through it. Whenever I felt my body become energized in this way, I would feel quite uncomfortable until I put my hands together, and when I put them together not only did the discomfort vanish, but I felt a deep sense of contentment. Once I put my hands together, the scattered waves of energy would blend together and would flow rhythmically through my arms.

Later when I began healing, I found the same phenomenon occurred, but the energy I experienced was more powerful. I felt my breath was coming from the left side of my body, and this coincided with unusual sensations which I felt on my left side as well. I discovered that the discomfort I experienced during prayer, which was alleviated when I put my hands together, was also alleviated when I touched my patient with both hands during laying on of hands. What I had unknowingly discovered is what I now call polarization.

Human Magnetism

As we know, the human body functions like an electric circuit. Energy flows through the nerves of the physical body causing a slight magnetic effect which results in a weak polarization. One side of the physical body has a weak positive charge, while the opposite side has a weak negative charge. This explains why healers feel different sensations on different sides of their body when it is polarized. This magnetic effect usually goes unnoticed and its importance in healing has been generally overlooked. However, when the healer opens his chakras through prayer, proper breathing and meditation and then channels prana through them, when he opens his heart and transmutes his desires into love, then the weak magnetic effect is transformed into a formidable tool for healing.

The magnetic energy generated through polarization must go somewhere, otherwise it becomes jammed at the nerve endings, many of which are located in the extremities: the hands and feet. This jamming causes the ache I mentioned earlier. As a rule magnetic energy travels in one direction, through the positive pole only. It behaves in the same way electrons do in an iron magnet, lining up in one direction in neat rows like soldiers. One side of the healer's polarized body acts as the positive pole asserting energy, while the other side acts as the negative pole and attracts healing energy from the higher planes.

When the body becomes polarized in this way, it is a clear indication large amounts of prana are available and it is ready to be focused on someone through the positive magnetic pole. For right handed people the positive pole would be the right hand, and the negative pole would be the left hand. For left handed people it would be reversed.

Direct Magnetic Healing

When the body is polarized and the heart chakra is sufficiently open, it acts like a vacuum pump. It pulls energy from the other chakras and transmutes it into the exact healing frequency your patient needs. Therefore, to heal through polarization you must open the heart chakra as much as possible. This can be done by using a combination of techniques which you already have learned. I suggest you heal by polarization after you have completed vibrational healing while your heart chakra is open, and you are projecting energy through it. It is important to understand that your success in polarization is dependent on your ability to work from the heart chakra. Polarization can be used separately if you have a limited time to perform laying on of hands, or it can be used along with other healing techniques during a complete healing session. In either case if you decide to use it, you must begin by breathing Yogically for a few moments. When you are sufficiently relaxed, then mentally affirm, "I am now deeply relaxed, and I am an open channel for healing energy." Then go into the alpha/theta state using one of the techniques you learned earlier. Once you are in the alpha/theta state, stimulate your heart chakra by paying attention to it and breathing from it. Once the chakra is stimulated it will open up and will become a channel for healing energy. When the chakra is open enough and a sufficient quantity of healing energy in the form of love and compassion is flowing through it, you will be able to think from the heart. While you are thinking from the heart and you feel healing energy coming through it, bring your attention to your hands. When you feel them begin to ache and you feel the desire to put your hands together, you will know that your physical body is polarized and magnetic energy is flowing through it. At that moment mentally affirm, "I am polarized and magnetic energy is flowing through me." Then spread your hands apart while keeping them on your patient's body (your hands should not be touching during polarization), and feel the rhythmic waves of energy flowing through them into your patient. Spend about five minutes healing through polarization, and keep working until you are satisfied the energy has had a healing effect. I have found I get the best results with polarization if I begin using it after I have achieved the vibrational state when I am working directly on the diseased area of my patient's body.

When you are satisfied with the effect polarization has had on your patient, move into one of the variations of polarization which are explained later in this chapter, or move into one of the other healing techniques you already know.

Staying Polarized

When your body is polarized, healing energy rhythmically flows through your masculine (positively charged) hand. It is important not to interfere with its rhythm. This can be difficult because there is an unconscious desire to synchronize the rhythm of the breath with any other physical rhythm which comes into consciousness. This is a trap which you must avoid because you will accomplish nothing through synchronization except depolarization. You can avoid synchronization by keeping your attention on your hands and off your breath. It is all right to observe the energy flowing through your hands with your unconscious mind, but you must avoid stimulating it consciously as well.

Stroking and Polarization

Stroking movements are very effective in healing when the body is polarized. They combine rhythmic hand movements, the breath, and magnetic energy, generated through polarization. When you begin using stroking, you will have to lift your hands from your patient's physical body and work in his etheric aura. You should begin using stroking movements while you are working on the diseased area of your patient's body before you return to the head. When you are ready to use the stroking variation, open your eyes (keep them unfocused), lift your hands from your patient's physical body and find the surface of his etheric aura with your masculine hand. On your next exhalation push downward with your positively charged hand like you were depressing a strong spring. Keep your other hand at shoulder level with your palm up. (See plate) Complete the exhalation as your positively charged hand reaches your patient's physical body. Each time you press downward, you should feel the rhythmic flow of energy coming from your negatively charged arm through your positively charged arm and into your patient's body. Keep breathing without separation between inhalation and exhalation, and continue with this technique until you feel the energy being absorbed by your patient. Once your patient begins absorbing the energy being projected through your hand, visualize it as a ray of energy in the appropriate healing color. Make sure the color you project is clear and bright. Then take two minutes to visualize the diseased tissue being transformed into perfect health.

Circular Passes

Another variation of polarization involves rhythmic circular passes which are made within your patient's aura above the diseased area. After you have polarized your body and you have completed working on the diseased tissue through polarization, lift your masculine hand from the surface of your patient's body (keeping it within his etheric aura), and hold your feminine hand at shoulder level with the palm up. (See plate) Then begin making slow, circular hand motions about three inches above the diseased tissue with your positively charged hand. Keep your hand flat, with your palm down while you are circling the problem area, and at the same time breathe deeply and slowly. The circles should always be made in a clockwise direction. Your breathing should be slightly forced, as if under pressure. As you make the circular passes, pay attention to the palm of your hand, and feel the energy flowing rhythmically through it. Then begin making the motions more

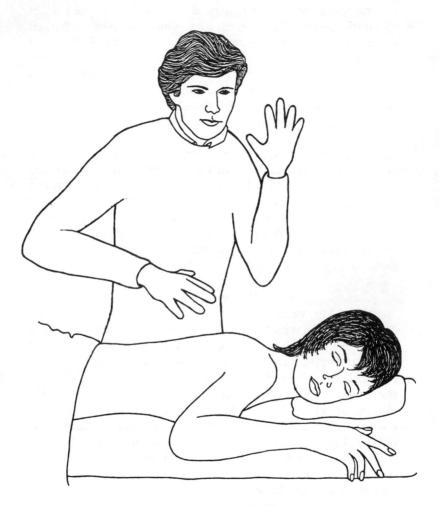

Plate 9: Stroking and Polarization

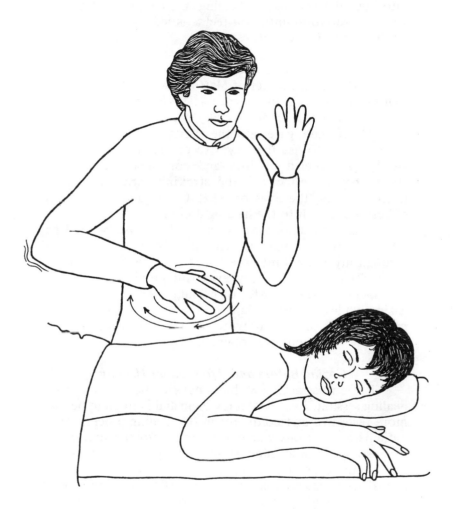

Plate 10: Hand in Circular Motion

rapid and visualize a colored ray of energy flowing from
your hand into your patient's aura. Feel it working its way
into the diseased tissue, healing it completely. Continue
with this variation until you feel satisfied the healing energy
has had a positive effect.

Gazing

In the sixth chapter of Matthew we are told that "the
Light of the body is in the eye . . ."[61] People who are magnetic or charismatic are usually admired because of the
strength of their gaze and the clarity of their eyes. They
have learned to use their eyes to project prana. A strong,
steady gaze fueled by love and compassion can have a
strong healing effect. In the stroking variations we are
learning, using the eyes or what I call gazing, can be an
effective addition to the healing process.

Gazing does not mean staring; when I use gazing I pay
attention to my patient without concentrating. I look
through my patient into the diseased tissue. Prana which is
being focused through my eyes will provide extra power
and facilitate the transfer of healing energy. You can use
gazing while you are making strokes or passes in a circular
motion or in pressing downward. You can use it anytime
you work with your eyes open.

Gazing Before and After Direct Healing

I often use gazing with my patients before and after a
healing session. I use it to relax them and help them become
more receptive and confident in the healing process. Many
patients are nervous when they arrrive for healing, simply
because spiritual healing is something new to them. Of
course, there are many other causes for anxiety. Regardless of what causes anxiety, it inhibits the healing process.
It would be ideal if the healer could begin healing and
relaxing his patient before the healing session begins. Gazing
gives the healer a tool to do just that. Some healers project
healing energy to their patients by gazing at them as soon
as they meet them. I have used gazing since I began doing

spiritual healing. Even while I am being introduced to my patient I use gazing; it has a very soothing effect on him. I have found that gazing affects me as well. It often leads me into an altered state of consciousness prior to the start of laying on of hands. Many times by simply gazing, I feel so much energy being channeled into the physical environment that the room itself becomes charged with energy, and the atmosphere becomes electrified.

During the initial introduction while I am explaining spiritual healing to my patient, I use gazing, often combining it with different forms of absentee healing. Since the eyes are unfocused in gazing, it is possible to remain conscious, and I can talk to my patient while I am projecting healing energy to him through my unconscious mind.

Sometimes a new patient will be so nervous that gazing prior to the healing session is ineffective in alleviating his tension. In cases like that, I have found gazing after the direct healing session is over can be effective. No matter how nervous a patient is, after the session he tends to relax. He feels the same way a student feels when final exams are over. Regardless of whether he passed or failed, the ordeal is over and there is nothing more to fear. In these cases I use gazing after I have finished laying on of hands. The patient's anxiety is rarely a chronic problem. Once the patient gets used to the healing process he invariably becomes more receptive and trusting.

Gazing can go beyond being a technique reserved for healing. It can become a vehicle of self-expression. It is the most efficient way to transmit prana into the environment; because of its magnetic effect it draws people to you and deepens your existing relationships.

Chakra Cleansing

Gazing and stroking are essential elements of chakra cleansing. Some healers use chakra cleansing as an integral part of each healing session. It can be used along with polarization after you have finished working on the diseased area, and after you have used the variations you just learned.

Chakra cleansing is useful in keeping your patient's chakras open, balanced and functioning properly. It has a beneficial effect on the entire subtle energy system. You always begin chakra cleansing with the seventh chakra and work downwards ending with the first chakra.

Begin with your eyes open and unfocused. With your masculine hand above his seventh chakra, find the surface of your patient's etheric aura. Then press downward while exhaling forcibly until you reach the surface of his physical body. Then inhale deeply without separation between inhalation and exhalation. Repeat this procedure three times, breathing out on each depression and breathing in as you return to the surface of his etheric aura. Your negatively charged hand should be held away from the patient with the palm up. This improves your receptivity to healing energy. After you make three strokes downward, begin the clockwise circular movement within the etheric aura above the chakra. Continue to breathe without separation between inhalation and exhalation, and keep thinking from your heart. As you gaze through the chakra, feel the blockages disappearing so the energy is no longer restricted. Repeat this technique with each of your patient's seven chakras. You shouldn't need more than twenty or thirty seconds to cleanse each chakra unless you discover a more severe problem in one of them. In that case, use polarization or one of its variations to project healing energy into the area. Later, you can complete the cleansing by resuming where you left off. Chakra cleansing, like chakra balancing and Yogic breathing, can be used as a preventative measure to maintain good health and prevent disease. Its effects are similar to those experienced in chakra balancing except they are stronger and the effects last longer. A person needn't be ill to benefit from chakra cleansing. You can practice it on anyone you like; your spouse, children, friends, etc.

As you can see, once the healer has achieved the state of polarization, he has several techniques at his disposal. He can work on the diseased area by touching the patient's body and allowing rhythmic pulsations to flow through his positively charged hand. He can work in the aura, using downward strokes or circular passes, and then he can combine stroking movements with gazing and absentee healing. Finally, he can do chakra cleansing.

The healer decides whether to use all of these techniques, or just one or two during each healing session. There is no set script; work intuitively and you will have the best results. When you are satisfied with what you have accomplished through polarization, bring your hands back to your patient's head. While working there you can use any of the techniques or combination of techniques to complete the session. When you are satisfied with the session, remove your hands from your patient's head, sit for a few moments and allow your chakras to fully recharge. The patient should be allowed to remain quiet for a minute or two while you are recharging and while you are washing your hands to clear away any residual negativity. The best way to end a direct healing session is the same way you end an absentee healing session. Begin counting from 1 to 5, using the appropriate affirmations to bring you back to normal consciousness. When you reach the number 5, open your eyes. You will feel wide awake, perfectly relaxed, and better than you did before.

CHAPTER SIXTEEN

EMPATHETIC HEALING

In this chapter you are going to study empathetic healing, the third part of laying on of hands. You will learn to use it in combination with the direct healing and absentee healing techniques you learned earlier. Each direct healing you perform will be different, and you won't use every technique you know during a given session. The length of time you devote to each technique and its placement during a healing will differ as well. However, when you master empathetic healing you will find that all your healing techniques merge into one and you will no longer consciously participate in the healing process.

Although empathetic healing is the most important and powerful method of healing, I left it for last because it is the most difficult technique to explain and understand. It begins when the healer transcends the duality of "me you" and no longer sees himself as separate from his patient, but experiences his patient and himself as one. The healer's job is to act as a bridge which connects his patient with the All, the source of healing. In empathetic healing the healer transcends his separate identity and reunites with the I AM. The I AM then merges with the patient and acts as a channel for God's healing energy. The temporary loss of personal identity allows the healer to experience disease the same way his patient does (although in a temporary and far milder form). He temporarily feels his patient's feelings, experiences his patient's bodily sensations and shares his patient's thoughts. We can say with some justification that in empathetic healing, the healer becomes the patient and heals himself.

Empathy and Union
Union has never been an easy state to achieve, whether it is union with another person or with God. However, it is the most important element in empathetic healing. To achieve union it is essential to surrender and reunite with the I AM. Only when the healer surrenders can his human qualities be transmuted into Divine qualities; only when he surrenders can human love become agape love, and human consciousness becomes Divine consciousness, etc.

The Conditions for Healing Empathetically
Certain conditions must be met before the healer can surrender completely and make the jump into empathetic healing. The healer must learn to pay attention at all times. He achieves this by functioning regularly in the alpha/theta state. He must remember he is a multi-dimensional being with masculine and feminine characteristics, who functions on all planes simultaneously. Then he must "recollect" himself by putting together all the pieces of his scattered identity. From recollection he finds relationship by transmuting human love into agape love and sharing it with anyone who needs it. Finally, by embracing the gift of faith he learns to surrender, and achieves union first with God and then with his patient.

To achieve the state necessary for empathetic healing, the healer must become skilled in the art of transmutation. He must learn to transmute energy on all four levels into any frequency he needs, whenever he needs it. To do this, the healer must become a master of Pranayama. He must be able to control his subtle energy system by controlling his breath. If his breathing is imperfect, then his energy system will operate defectively and empathic healing will be impossible. The healer must have a relaxed mind which thinks—on command—either in pictures or remains empty and clear. The healer's physical body must be free of tension and his chakras must be open and balanced, ready to transmit vast amounts of prana to his patient. The healer must be able to polarize his energy system and he must be able to bring the central pranic vibration into consciousness. When all these conditions are met the healer will feel his conscious mind receding into the background. It is at this point that the I AM takes over, and it becomes possible to work empathetically. As you can see, the techniques you studied to this point are the prerequisites for empathetic healing. Only when you have mastered them will you be able to proceed to the final, most dramatic phase of healing. You will find that, "Beyond the world of matter; beyond the creative force of Brahma, there is the great non dual existence prevailing all and residing in all, taking their shapes as the personal God of every being . . ."[62]

Mastering Empathetic Healing

Empathetic healing must be preceded by the mastery of vibrational healing or polarization. Either of these two techniques can act as the starting point for working empathetically. When you have completed working either through vibration or polarization, you can begin empathetic healing by mentally affirming, "The presence of God is with us and we are one in Him." Then you must focus all your attention on your patient until you feel his feelings as your own. This should only take a few moments. You will experience at this time, a change in your breathing. Your breath and the breath of your patient will ebb and flow in the same rhythm, and with every breath you take, you will feel more connected to him. Some healers feel unusual sensations coming from their solar plexus when they perform empathetic healing, because it is from the solar plexus that we feel connected to people, places and things.

Merging With Your Patient

When you feel every movement of your patient's

heart as if it were your own, then you will feel yourself
drift out of your body, and you will feel yourself merging
with him. You can merge with your patient in two ways.
You can do it mentally or etherically. When it is soley your
mind or consciousness which is projected outside your
physical body, you will connect with your patient on the
mental plane, and the experience will be the same as in
mental projection. But when you project your etheric
body outside your physical body and you merge with your
patient's etheric body as well, you will become one with him
and you will be free from the restriction of your physical
body. It is in this way that you want to connect with your
patient in empathetic healing. You will begin by merging
etheric bodies, but with practice you can go much further.
You can merge with your patient's corresponding body on
each of the three higher levels; the etheric level, mental level
and spiritual level.

In its initial stages when the etheric body begins to
leave the confines of the physical body, the healer will often
feel himself drift upward, downward, or from side to side.
This is a partial projection and in itself is useful because
when the etheric body leaves the physical body, it is freed
from the control of the conscious mind and the All has
more direct contact with the patient. Moreover, the central
pranic vibration will grow stronger and more prana will
flow from your subtle energy system into your patient.

By leaving your body completely during empathetic
healing, the All is not blocked by any of the tensions,
doubts and fears which you have. There is no conscious
mind to interfere with his consciousness, and there is no
physical body to restrict the flow of prana. Thus the All
can work through you without restriction, and the work
will be the most direct and complete, often culminating
in spontaneous complete healing.

As a healer you must cultivate detachment by dividing
yourself into two parts. You must learn to think from the
heart, to heal from the heart and to project your consciousness to your patient while you allow the conscious

self, the objective mind and the ego to remain separate, relegated to the role of observer and occasionally to programmer.

The Patient's Attitude

In empathetic healing more than any other form of healing, the patient's attitude is important. If the patient is closed, anxious or untrusting, then the healer will be prevented from uniting completely with his patient. On the other hand, if the patient believes in the healing process, expects to be healed, and if he has sufficient faith in the healer, then empathetic healing will be possible and the probability of a spontaneous and complete healing is substantially increased.

For several months I worked on a female patient in her mid seventies who suffered from arthritis which caused her extreme pain, especially in her hip and lower back. My rapport with her was excellent and I was able to work empathetically with her for long periods of time. She was open enough for me to merge easily with her, and as a result I worked on her during my meditations while I was engaged in absentee healing. Because of her advanced age and the extent of her condition, we never achieved a complete physical healing. However, I was able to substantially reduce her level of pain. As a result she was able to sleep undisturbed, which for many years she was unable to do. She was also able to return to activities she had been forced to put aside because of her disability. I believe it was because of our excellent rapport and because of her openness that she benefited from empathetic healing.

In the case I just cited, empathetic healing was useful in relieving pain, but you should remember it is through empathetic healing, through union with God and with your patient that spontaneous healings can happen.

A Complete Empathetic Healing

In another case, a spontaneous healing resulted from empathetic healing. It occurred in one of my classes while

I demonstrated empathetic healing as part of the workshop curriculum. In October of 1981, I demonstrated on a young woman who volunteered to be my subject. I quote here from a letter I received from her on November 13, 1981:

> On September 11, 1981, I entered the New York University Hospital to have my tonsils removed. . . on the night before the operation a nodule was discovered on the upper left side of my lung. X-rays from three years prior to that discovery were compared to the current x-rays so the presence of the nodule was definitely confirmed in a front and side x-ray from New York University. The doctors had decided a Cat-scan would be necessary to obtain more information as to where this nodule was located and the consistency of it.
>
> Meanwhile I had been taking your Psychic Development class and had volunteered myself as your psychic healing participant in the third class session. This was two weeks after the discovery of the lung nodule. . . My scan had been cancelled due to failure of equipment and was postponed to October 16 from October 8. While under the scanner, the doctor in charge confirmed that nothing had shown up and the lung was clear.
>
> While I had been in the process of psychic healing, I had actually felt the warmth of the healing energy through me. In fact, the left side of my body (where the nodule was) even seemed to be floating in the air, while the right side was still on the couch. You had chosen the area without me telling you where the nodule was located.
>
> I firmly believe that a psychic healing actually occurred by the dizziness I felt afterwards. I'd like to thank you (and the Christ spirit that came through you because I know you don't take credit) for the healing. You probably saved me a painful and expensive operation and have helped me confirm my belief in psychic healing and the psychic, spiritual aspects of life.

Putting It All Together

A complete direct healing session is a synthesis of absentee and direct healing techniques which culminates in empathetic healing. When you are ready to perform a direct healing session with your patient, you should begin by explaining the techniques of laying on of hands with him while you are making him relaxed and comfortable. You can help your patient relax by having him lie down and leading him into the Yogic breath. Next, you should make yourself comfortable and begin breathing Yogically yourself. Then mentally affirm, "I am in the alpha level and my hands are becoming sensitive." When you are ready, make three complete passes through your patient's etheric aura with your hands. Keep your palms down and your fingers loosely extended. After your final pass, find the surface of your patient's etheric aura with your masculine hand. Use that hand to skim your patient's aura, and take the next few minutes to diagnose your patient's condition. When you are finished with his front, have your patient turn over and repeat the process with his back. If you discover any problems in his aura, project your consciousness inside the body and complete your diagnosis from inside the body.

When your diagnosis is complete, sit down at the head of your patient, close your eyes and resume the Yogic breathing. Feel yourself going deeper on each exhalation. Then mentally affirm, "I am a channel for healing, and healing energy is coming through me." Place your hands on your patient's head and let the Yogic breathing lead you into the vibrational state. Remember to pay attention to the rhythms of your body and allow your bodily rhythms to direct the rhythm of your breathing. Your breath should be slightly forced, and you should continue breathing without separation between inhalation and exhalation until you feel your hands vibrate and get hot. Once the vibration becomes self-sustaining you will be solidly in the vibrational state. Work on your patient's head using vibrational healing for about five minutes, and let the central pranic vibration supersede the initial vibration. Then move to the diseased area of your patient's body without disrupting the vibration. Remember to keep your hands apart. Once you have changed position, continue healing with this technique for three or four minutes. If absentee healing techniques appear spontaneously, use them along with vibrational healing.

When you are satisfied with the effects of vibrational healing, pay attention and breathe from your heart chakra. Mentally affirm, "I am polarized and magnetic energy is flowing through me." When you have stimulated your heart chakra sufficiently, your arms and hands will begin to ache and you will have a strong desire to put them together. These are signs that your body has become polarized. Spend the next five minutes healing through polarization and feel the rhythmic waves of energy flowing through your masculine hand into your patient. Work for the first two or three minutes using polarity exclusively. Then while your body remains polarized, visualize a ray of energy in the appropriate color flowing from your heart chakra into the diseased area of your patient's body. Feel your patient absorbing the ray of energy with gratitude.

After two or three minutes or when you are satisfied with the effects of polarity and chakra healing, lift your hands from your patient's body, open your eyes (keep them unfocused) and begin the stroking variations. Start by finding the surface of your patient's etheric aura with your masculine hand and on your next exhalation, push downward with your positively charged hand like you were depressing a strong spring. Keep your other hand at shoulder level with your palm up. Complete your exhalation as your positively charged hand reaches your patient's physical body. Once your patient begins absorbing the energy being projected through your hand, visualize the energy coming through your hand as a ray of energy in the appropriate healing color and feel your patient absorb it with gratitude. Take two minutes to heal through this variation. When you are finished, begin making clockwise circular passes with your masculine hand in your patient's etheric aura about three inches above your patient's physical body. Keep your hand flat with your palm down while you are circling the problem area, and at the same time breathe deeply and slowly. Your breathing should be slightly forced, as if under pressure. As you make the circular passes, pay attention to the palm of your hand and feel the energy rhythmically flowing through it. Then begin making the circular motions more rapid and visualize a colored ray of energy flowing from your hand into your patient's aura. Feel it working its way into the diseased tissue, healing it completely. Continue this variation for two or three minutes or until you feel satisfied the energy from your hand has had a healing effect. You can complete your work with polarization and stroking by cleansing your patient's chakras. Remember to begin with the seventh chakra and end with the first chakra.

After these variations, return to your patient's head and mentally affirm, "Every time I come to these levels of mind it makes it easier for me to go to deeper and healthier levels." Then count from 10 to 1 backwards and feel yourself going deeper. Next, mentally affirm, "The presence of God is with us and we are one in Him." Focus all your attention on your patient and empathize with him until you feel his feelings as your own. At your deep level of consciousness this should take only a few moments. After a few moments you will notice a change in your breathing. Your breath and the breath of your patient will ebb and flow in the same rhythm, and with every breath you take you will feel more connected to him. When you feel every movement of your patient's heart as if it were your own, then feel yourself drifting out of your body and feel yourself merging with him. When you are in union with him, all your techniques will merge into one and you will be able to work empathetically with him. Continue working empathetically with him for five minutes or until you are satisfied.

When you are satisfied with the session, remove your hands from your patient's head, sit for a few moments and allow your chakras to recharge. While you are recharging mentally affirm, "Every time I act as a channel for healing, not only is my patient healed, but I am healed as well." When you feel your chakras are completely recharged, begin counting from 1 to 5 slowly. When you reach the number 5, open your eyes. You will feel wide awake, perfectly relaxed and better than you did before. Finally, immerse your hands in cold running water three times to remove any residual negativity you might have picked up during the healing session. When you are finished, return to your patient and while you discuss your patient's experience during the healing session, enjoy the effects that empathetic healing has had on you and on your patient.

CHAPTER SEVENTEEN

GOING BEYOND THE EGO

Two of the questions which invariably come up in spiritual healing are: what purpose does the ego play during healing, and how does the healer protect his ego from negativity during an absentee healing session or during laying on of hands. I'd like to address those two questions in this chapter. Excluding contagious diseases, it is unheard of for a healer to pick up any disease from his patient which directly affects his physical body. However, in both laying on of hands and in absentee healing, the healer is projecting his consciousness inside his patient; he is making contact with his patient on the mental and etheric planes and although there can't be any direct transfer of physical disease, it is possible for the healer to pick up negativity mentally in the form of negative thoughts and images, and emotionally in the form of negative feelings. There should be no problem if the healer remains detached, if the healer's ego stays out of the way, if he remembers he is only the channel for healing. However, if the healer's ego, his lower conscious self inserts itself into the healing process, then there can be a problem. The lower self has no function in healing, and it should move aside as soon as healing begins. It should move aside in deference to the I AM which alone acts as the channel for Divine healing energy. In short, only if the lower self, the ego, usurps God's function attempting to perform healing on its own will there be a problem.

Transmuting Negativity on the Mental Plane

From the beginning I have stressed that the healer is a channel. God is the healer. If you remember this fact, there shouldn't be any problems. If a problem does arise, and you begin experiencing negativity while practicing absentee healing, stop the healing at once and use the "Cancel, cancel" technique you learned in Chapter Three. If a negative emotional response has already occurred, immediately begin reprogramming. Begin by using the techniques you learned earlier and go into the alpha/theta level. When you feel deeply relaxed, when your eyes are unfocused and you are thinking in pictures, mentally affirm, "Negativity has no affect on me at any level of mind." Keep repeating this affirmation until you've regained your composure and the negativity has dissipated. Then use positive affirmations to reinforce your positive mental state. Mentally affirm, "Every time I overcome negativity, I grow stronger", and then, "I am a child of God, a channel for His love and power." Continue these affirmations as long as you feel they are necessary. Add a few of your own if you like. Finally, let the Yogic breath lead you into a brief meditation. During your meditation, create positive images in your mind to complete the programming. If you resist the initial anxiety and use the techniques you already know, you can turn a negative experience into a positive one.

The Problem of the Ego in Healing

When I began healing, I sometimes overstepped my bounds by trying too hard. I believed I could improve on God's technique by pushing my ego into places where it didn't belong. I knew each time my ego stepped in where it didn't belong, because the experience was painful. Since negativity hurts and I didn't like it, I was forced to find ways to prevent the pain. I intuitively knew that only if I transcended ego would I become an effective channel for healing. But my initial efforts to overcome the ego failed. I fould the ego is tricky and doesn't like to be ignored or put on the shelf. Notwithstanding my best efforts, my ego could sometimes find ingenious ways to insert itself into the healing process. This continued until I began listening to the I AM, and became detached. Transcendence came when I put my will in accord with God's will. It might help you to know a person can only be attached to those things which he fears or desires. I found a direct assault on fears and desires was useless because "I" was the one making the assault and "I" was the one being assaulted. Trying to change in this way was counterproductive because the "I" in both cases was the ego, and the desire for self-improvement was nothing more than a ploy which the ego used to confuse me so it could retain its preeminent position. But I knew the ego had to move aside at least during a healing session to make room for the Divine energy which did the healing.

Transcending Ego

My experiences led me to the conclusion that my attempts to dispose the ego were fruitless. I learned the ego is preeminent on the earth plane. It can never be overcome by force; it can only be transcended and for that we need help. This help cannot come from another person; at least not directly. It can only come from our higher self, the I AM. Only the I AM is powerful enough and clever enough to overpower and outwit the ego. It alone can push the ego from its loftly position. The I AM overcomes ego, not through force, and it doesn't attack the ego, because a healthy ego is necessary in everyday life. It transcends the ego by bringing a person into a higher level of consciousness. At this new level, the power of *karma* (cause and effect) is transcended and the ego is forced to submit to its new partner, the I AM.

The I AM and Union

What you will eventually discover when you recognize the I AM is that you are the I AM. The I AM is your heart speaking to you through your intuition and through your conscience. When you listen to it long enough, it will begin

to influence you in a host of ways. At first, it will serve
you as an advisor, then as a partner and finally as a friend.
When the friendship has become intimate and trust abides,
a miraculous thing happens. You become the I AM. You
learn at last that you have always been the I AM. You
realize you are not the ego nor are you the personality.
These were masks you mistakenly identified with, and in
time you came to believe you were nothing more than
these masks. However, once you realize you are more than
ego and more than personality, your transformation will
begin. You will realize that separation, your belief you are
separate from the rest of creation, is an illusion. Once you
go beyond separation and see that you are part of everything else, you will find yourself in union with all other
life forms. The I AM will then flow through you into each
one of them, healing them on all levels. In time, your personality will be transformed, becoming deeply enriched,
becoming a Divine tool serving the I AM, becoming the
temple of God's healing spirit.

> . . . Had not my soul's, thy conduit, pipes stoppes
>   been
> With mud, what ravishment wouldst thou convey?
> Let grace's golden spade dig till the spring
> Of tears arise, and clears this filth away.
> Lord; let thy spirit raise my sighings till
> These pipes my soul do with thy sweetness fill...63

Separation and Disease
Separation is not the natural state of being for anyone,
but it has become the normal state for the vast majority of
people today. It is a state of disease because in one way or
another, each person who experiences separation seeks
reunion with the I AM. If an individual fails in his attempts
to reunite, then he will seek union with just about anything.
This is the origin of all forms of addictive behavior. Separation causes disease; disease is painful. People in pain seek
solace and comfort; if they can't find it on the inner realms

they seek it in the physical world. They seek union in their work through sex, overeating, or even drugs, through an endless variety of addictive activities. What's important is the root cause of these addictions is separation from the I AM, from the self. As the Bible says, "For what is a man profited, if he shall gain the whole world, but lose his own soul?"

Reunion and Self-Realization
Reunion through self-realization has always been the goal of the most ardent souls; the goal of those seeking an end to disease on every level. Many routes lead to reunion with the I AM, and the way for one person cannot always be the way for another. Karma, temperament and a host of other factors determine each person's particular path or *dharma*. Because of the differences among people, the ancient Yogis developed eight schools of Yoga. Individual temperament determines which of these paths will lead a person into union. In the *Bhagavad Gita*, the Lord Krishna explains that Karma Yoga, the path of action and service, is for those who work; the path of action leads back to union. He explains that right action, selfless action or service, springs not from ego but from the "supreme spirit" the I AM. In healing we perform our service selflessly. We perform Karma Yoga by acting as channels, letting the All heal through the I AM within us.

I am often asked: what is the most direct route to union and self-realization? The answer is: by serving others. In healing, we serve by merging with the All, and then with the patient. We act as channels and in the process we transcend the ego. Transcendence and the union which results from transcendence is so joyful that afterwards the healer seeks transcendence and union in all his relationships. When this happens the process of realization will be securely on its way. Direct experience of God's power through healing and the experience of His spirit through union with the I AM will lead a person into a greater understanding of God's love, power, and a greater desire to experience more of Him, more often. For those who are looking for the "way", I encourage you to begin healing. It might be part of your dharma, your true path.

Finding My Dharma

A person's life path, his dharma, is a roadmap which he must follow if he hopes to find meaning and happiness in his life. In my life, I turned my back on true dharma for years. My initial fear of being different, of hearing a "different drummer" caused me to deny and neglect my path and my true work. My fear of being myself and accepting myself and my dharma pushed me in many useless directions before my frustration forced me to stop. While I traveled with my teacher, I repeatedly refused to transcend ego, to listen to and obey my "inner guide". I would indulge my ego rather than follow the guidance of the I AM. The result was frustration and fear. It was only after my teacher told me to leave that I began to face the conflicts between my ego and the I AM.

A Parable

As I was leaving, he told me a story which I have never forgotten. The story begins when a young man meets his teacher for the first time. He asks the teacher if he will take him on as a student. The teacher accepts the student but on one condition; before they begin the young man must go sailing with the teacher. The young man excitedly agrees. The next day the two leave the safety of the harbor and they sail away together. Their voyage begins slowly and uneventfully, but soon the wind picks up and they go faster and farther with each passing day. As they race through the waves, the student forgets about his past unhappiness. He is entranced by the excitement and the adventure. He sees new places and experiences new things. He is happy for awhile. He even forgets his original quest, but something within him remains unsatisfied. And soon his longing returns, this time with greater urgency. As the days pass the teacher sees the young man's discomfort grow. Finally, on a calm day far from land, the teacher folds the sail away and allows the boat to drift on its own. Then he asks the young man, "Why did you come on this trip with me? Was it for the excitement only or was there something else, something deep within you which pulled you to me? Was it adventure and excitement which forced you to forsake everything, or was it your inner yearning for reunion which led you to me?" The young man didn't answer. "Sailing is not part of the teaching" the old man continued. "I brought you here so that the teaching could begin. I had to take you away from your comforts and your bad habits. I brought you here so that you could forget your old attachments and leave them behind. You had to learn that the things you left behind weren't essential. Your happiness didn't depend upon them. But still you're not satisfied, and that's because you are still "you". The problem remains. The problem is you! To reach your goal, something in you must change. The undisputed reign of your ego must end so the real you, the I AM can emerge. Realization, the thing you desire most, has always been attained in this way. It can only be achieved through surrender.

Now look out to the sea. You are like the sea; your ego keeps you separate from yourself. The sea is everything; the sea is you, the All, everything that ever was or ever will be. You must leave your ego behind and submerge yourself in the sea. You must surrender to it and only then will you transcend the pain of separation, and achieve union and peace."

The student hesitated for a moment and then replied, "I want what you have, I want to be free." Like a flash, the older man grabbed the youth and heaved him overboard. The young man landed in the water, but immediately began splashing wildly. In his panic he forgot everything the old man had told him, and he tried desperately to swim back to the boat.

At first the teacher cried out. "Have faith, don't give in to your fear." But the young man couldn't hear him. He thought only of saving himself. Finally, he managed to get a grip on the side of the boat and he wouldn't let go. The teacher reluctantly helped the youth back into the boat, and for while the young man lay exhausted in the bottom of the boat. For a long time they said nothing to one another while the teacher sat at the tiller and steered the boat home. After a time, they arrived at the harbor and the teacher docked the boat. At last they spoke. The teacher said, "There are many things in this world to learn, but they are only preparation. The goal of all learning is reunion and self-realization. Reunion can only be achieved through surrender, and that is ultimately the only thing worth having. You have learned many things, but not that. You are still a slave to your ego. Your fears and desires still control you. You learn very quickly, but your goal still eludes you. You are still "you". Now you must go. You don't need me anymore. Go back to the world and let the world be your teacher. Perhaps you will find your 'self' there."

I didn't say anything after that. All I could do was leave. I saw that story for what it was; a metaphor of our relationship. Years later, my dharma became clear and through my work in healing I surrendered to the I AM and achieved my goal. Self-realization came when I acknowledged my true dharma and had the courage to follow it. I discovered that self-realization came through service and God provided me with the way, by using me as a channel for healing.

CHAPTER EIGHTEEN

A DAILY REGIMEN FOR GOOD HEALTH

Total health is the goal of spiritual healing, and total health is a return to harmony and balance as we have discovered. So far we have learned techniques which will help us achieve harmony and balance in our higher bodies and in our subtle energy system. Harmony and balance on the higher planes is in turn transmuted into good health on the physical plane. But we should not become myopic and think that by working on the higher planes we can disregard the importance of our relationship to the physical environment. Indeed, the relationship a person has with the physical world must be brought into balance if good health is to be achieved, and must remain in balance if one hopes to stay in good health once it has been restored. The purpose of this chapter is to suggest a daily regimen which will keep each of you in harmony with the physical environment, and which will keep you in good health once it has been restored through the techniques of spiritual healing.

As we already know, the life process is never static; life flows rhythmically either in the direction of health or in the direction of disease. As a consequence, none of us can afford to become complacent about our good health. What we do and even what we neglect to do on the physical plane can have a significant influence on our physical health and on the health of our higher bodies (remember disease is transmuted to the adjacent body regardless of where the disease condition originates). It should be clear then, that

185

our actions and reactions to the physical world and our total relationship to it in the form of eating, sleeping, rest, work, etc. can contribute significantly to our state of health.

Disease as we experience it in the physical plane is normally a symptom of deeper problems which can be traced back to the higher planes. Once negative patterns have taken root in the physical body, they can have an inertia of their own, and they can have a negative impact on the health of our higher bodies. This kind of negative conditioning creates negative patterns, and they in turn create fertile ground for negative attitudes, negative human relationships, and a negative relationship to stress. These negative patterns must be transmuted into positive attitudes and relationships if total health is to be permanently achieved.

Is Stress the Enemy
For a moment, let's consider the subject of stress. For years stress has been maligned as the unseen enemy of good health and the harbinger of disease. But is it really stress which is our enemy, or is it our attitude to stress which is to blame? Let's look at some research recently done on the chemical ACTH (adrenocortico-tropic hormone). It is considered by many experts on learning to be the most important hormone your body can produce. A number of experiments have recently revealed that when stress was created in laboratory animals, so was ACTH. In addition, researchers discovered that ACTH in laboratory animals produced new neuron links in their brains. Neuron links are tiny bridges in the brain which connect brain cells, and these little bridges are the keys to learning. The more neuron links the rats had, the faster they learned and the more they retained. The same holds true for human beings. By being the agent of positive change, stress in these experiments revealed its true nature is not singular but polar. From experiments such as these, we have learned that stressful situations are inherently subjective. A person's perception determines whether a stressful situation will be

viewed as positive or negative. It is not stress, but a person's reaction to stress and negativity which is always the real issue in the struggle between good health and disease. By accepting your innate responsibility for your health and well-being, you will begin to appreciate the significance of your actions and reactions to your overall state of health. To help insure your continued good health, you must take your responsibility seriously and take prudent steps which will promote health in both your internal and external environments, and thereafter practice a daily program which will promote the proper flow of energy through your subtle energy system and maintain the proper relationship between your four bodies. In this chapter I will outline a daily program which I believe will keep you in good health once it has been restored.

Regularity

Over two thousand years ago Hippocrates advised those around him that regularity was an indicator of good health, and that irregularity both in bodily functions or personal habits promoted disease. Gay Luce tells us that, "A healthy person lives in harmony with his environment." She goes on to say, "It is abundantly clear that healthy human beings are not only internally rhythmic; they are synchronized with their environment."[64]

The overwhelming evidence seems to point to the importance of rhythmicity to good health, and any program designed to promote good health must promote regularity. I suggest you begin your daily program of health by examining your lifestyle; the way you live, conduct your affairs and relate to others. Check to see if there is a built in irregularity which in itself could be the breeding ground for disease. You can do this simply by spending a week carrying a small pad and pen with you and keeping track of the different activities you take part in during the day. Take note of when you go to sleep and when you wake up, when you eat regular meals, when you snack, when you work and when you rest, and the different kinds of activities

you perform while working and resting. You should even
note how much time you spend alone and how much time
you spend with your friends or family. Keep a separate
column where you register comments beside each phase of
activity, and expecially make notes and observations about
how you felt at the end of each activity and again at the
end of each day.

   I think after a day or two you will begin to see patterns emerge, and you will find your well-being is directly
tied to the kinds of activities you perform and their regularity. For example, you may discover that when you disrupt
your normal patterns of sleep by staying out late, you feel
anxious the next day; you may find that on days where
your routine is regular and predictable you sleep better
and wake up more refreshed the next morning. In general,
I think you will find when you follow a regular routine,
you function better, feel better and stay healthier.

   The relationship between rhythmicity, health and
even productivity has not escaped close scientific scrutiny.
It has been studied not only in the laboratory, but in the
field through the observation and investigation of critical
national and world events. The links between the outside
world and a person's internal rhythms are called *zeitgebers*
(German for time givers). These outside triggers (often
rhythms themselves such as the day-night cycle) cue the
body clocks within us and can even upset them. Food and
drink are powerful *zeitgebers*, so is stress. Our internal
clocks and rhythms will also be affected by a break in daily
rhythm, such as changing work hours. Such disruption in
daily rhythms can play havoc on our delicate internal
machinery, and with a worker's health and overall ability
to function. Scientists have an example of just this kind of
disruption in the accident at the Three Mile Island nuclear
facility where it was normal for the workers to change shifts
every week. This would mean their internal clocks were out
of sync during most of the hours they were at work. If there
is a direct relationship between productivity, health and
rhythm, researchers would expect to find that the workers

would be disoriented, have memory lapses, impaired judgement and difficulty in paying attention. They would also be expected to react lethargically during a crisis if their rhythms had been disrupted. The investigation into the causes of the accident showed that in the hours preceding the accident (which incidentally occurred at 4 AM) there was evidence in the logbook of small errors in meter reading and interpreting data made by the workers on shift change.

Jet lag is another *zeitgeber* which is known to disrupt a person's internal rhythms and can impair efficiency and judgement. In 1956 John Foster Dulles, the secretary of state under president Eisenhower, flew to Egypt to conduct negotiations with the Egyptian government on the construction of the Aswan Dam. Subsequent to his arrival the talks broke down; this blunder in foreign policy had the effect of pushing the Egyptians into the arms of the Soviets. It is interesting to note that Dulles entered the meeting right after deplaning, and later attributed his poor judgement to jet lag.

Chemical Rest

It was Hippocrates who said that regularity was the first step in maintaining good health. He believed as many modern healers do that the second step was rest; not only physical rest, but chemical rest which he considered even more important. The chemical rest he prescribed could only be achieved by withholding food from the body and allowing it to cleanse itself, and to discharge the waste products that had built up within it. The rest he spoke of need not be anything as radical as a long and complete fast from food. Instead, short, rhythmic fasts are prescribed more often and are more desirable since they can become part of a person's daily regimen. The first rest that should become a regular part of your health program is the rest between dinner and breakfast. Studies have shown that the evening is not the best time for the body to digest and assimilate large amounts of food. In a study conducted several years ago by Dr. Grans Halberg at the University of Minnesota, six volunteers were given a single meal at breakfast time consisting of two thousand calories. The volunteers continued on this schedule for one week. In the second week of the experiment, the same volunteers were given an identical meal with only one difference. Instead of eating it at breakfast time, they ate it in the evening at dinner time. On the breakfast schedule all six volunteers lost weight. However, on the dinner-only schedule, four of the six gained weight while the remaining two, even though losing weight, lost less than they did on the breakfast-only regimen.[65] It makes sense to eat less in the evening when the body doesn't need so many calories. By eating less in the evening, the physical body not only gets a chance to sleep, but to have a short chemical rest which it can use to throw off toxins.

Undernutrition

You can take the chemical rest one step further with the possibility of even more startling results. In the 1940's professors A. H. Carlson and his colleague F. Holzel conducted experiments on rats to study the effects of intermittent fasting on their life span. They provided the rats with a high nutrition, high quality diet and the rats were permitted to eat as much as they wanted. The one wrinkle was that each of the rat groups participating in the experiment were fasted in different sequences. The first group was fasted completely every second day; the second group was fasted every third day, and the third group went without food every fourth day. The control group ate the same diet as the other three groups, except there was no periodic fasting imposed. In the control group, the maximum life span recorded was 800 days, while in the fasted groups the life span recorded ranged on the average between 1,000 and 1,100 days, a 20% to 30% extension of life span.[66]

Further studies of dietary restriction have yielded other noteworthy results. For example, a number of studies have indicated that undernutrition (caloric restriction) without malnutrition in rats produced chemically younger rats than their chronological age would indicate. Experiments conducted at UCLA by Dr. Richard Weindruch and Roy Walford have shown that dietary restriction has a rejuvenating effect on the immunological system . . . with advanced age the immunological system's ability to distinguish between self and foreign bodies becomes blurred, and the aging process is characterized by anti-self reactions as well as a weakened ability to combat foreign and toxic substances. It can decline as much as 20-30% of the youthful peak in old age. Dietary restriction counteracts both of these trends. In experiments with mature rats, dietary restriction beginning in adulthood actually leads to a dramatic and substantial rejuvenation of the immunological system. The tendency of anti self-reactions is also substantially reduced. What other effects does caloric undernutrition have? Preliminary work with laboratory animals indicates diseases such as cancer, cataracts, skin dryness, kidney and heart disease are found less frequently in animals raised under caloric restriction than rats raised normally. In addition, not only is there less disease, but when it does appear, it appears later in life.[67]

Good Nutrition

Caloric restriction practiced regularly (rhythmically), clearly translates into good health. Not only does rhythmic fasting promote good health, but eating the right kinds of food can play an important part in maintaining good health. Dr. Henry Bieler, a pioneer in the study of nutrition tells us that blood, besides fueling the physical body, can do much more for us. It can be our best medicine. Dr. Bieler is a strong proponent of good nutrition as a combatant against disease. He makes a strong case by citing the often overlooked truth that 80-85% of all types of human disease are self-limiting; they must run their course and when they are finished the patient recovers.[68] On the other side, since the 1970's, food is being increasingly discussed in terms of risk/benefit. This is not surprising since six of the nation's leading killers: heart disease, cancer, stroke, hypertension, diabetes, and arteriuscleriosis are directly linked to diet.[69]

Even with the abundance of foodstuffs, Americans rarely take advantage of the good nutritional food available. As Dr. Henry Beigler points out: Americans subsist "on lifeless, overprocessed, insecticide-sprayed food; saturated with toxic matter from such stimulators as coffee, tea, alcohol, chocolate, sweetened cola drinks; medicated with stimulating pep-up drugs, men and women whose low state of health just barely keeps them alive." Junk foods (foods with little or no nutritional value) account for about 26% of the average caloric intake of Americans today. Dr. Donald Davis of the University of California at Irvine conducted an experiment in which he fed a select group of rats a diet modeled on the standard American diet. The diet included white enriched bread, sugar, eggs, milk, ground beef, cabbage, potatoes, tomatoes, oranges, apples, bananas and coffee. The control group was fed a diet of equal caloric content made up solely of Purina Cat Chow. Compared to the rats on the Purina Cat Chow diet, the rats on the American diet fared quite poorly, falling far behind the control group in both overall health and growth rates. As you can see, any program designed to maintain and promote good health must consider the role of proper nutrition. Proper nutrition becomes even more of a consideration when you adopt a program of caloric restriction. With fewer calories available, what you eat must have the maximum nutritional value possible.

Even though individual needs differ, it would be wise to consider what the average human being really needs in his diet to stay healthy, and what he could do without or what is downright harmful to himself. Jane Brody tells us, "Homo sapiens evolved on a diet rich in complex carbohydrates and fiber (from starchy food, vegetables and fruits) and low in animal protein."[71] This is a far cry from the modern American diet which is high in meat, full of processed sweets, low in fiber, full of nutritionally empty fats, sugar and alcohol. It is essential for anyone concerned about restoring good health or maintaining good health to take stock of what he puts into his body, and then take measures to remove those elements which are clearly harmful or become harmful because they are taken in excess. On the other side, we must take care to provide the essential nutrients, vitamins or molecules our physical body needs. Ortho molecular nutritionists have discovered that what your diet lacks can have just as big an impact on your health as what you over-indulge in. For example, hypoglycemia (low blood sugar) is capable of producing a wide range of psychiatric symtoms, including psychosis.

Let's Eat Right
In this chapter I will give you only the bare outlines of what enlightened researchers tell us makes good nutritional sense. You must take it from there by educating yourself and paying attention, i.e. listening to your body. You must come up with a nutritional program which fits your lifestyle and works for you. Ther are several guidelines which can apply to all of us. Everyone's diet should consist of a wide variety of foods, and no one food should make up more than 25% of a day's caloric intake. If it does, chances are you are depriving your body of some necessary nutrients. So-called fortified foods and supplements are no substitute for whole, natural foods. Chemical additives should be consistently avoided. So should salt. Decrease your consumption of processed sugars. Limit your intake of high fat foods, especially foods high in animal fats. Eat your fruits and vegetables raw as often as possible (cooking destroys nutrients). Eat fruits and vegetables when they are at the height of their nutritional value. To do this, focus on fruits and vegetables grown locally and eat them during their natural season. Finally, buy food often, so your conscious choice of what to buy and eat comes out of bodily need. By listening to your body, you will select foods which contain the nutrients your body requires.

Nutrients provide us with the energy and building materials necessary to sustain us physically. Our physical body is made up mostly of protein, which is widely considered to be the most important nutrient. But Americans need far less protein than they normally consume. The problem with consuming too much protein is that most of the protein-rich food we eat is packed with fat and calories, far more than most people need, and far more than you should have to stay healthy. Instead, it would be wise to substitute complex carbohydrates, which are often excellent sources of protein, for animal protein, which is full of artery-clogging fats. It has been found that vegetarians who substitute plant proteins for animal proteins have lower blood pressure and far less fat and cholesterol in their system than Americans who eat meat.

Proteins are made up of amino acids. There are twenty two amino acids found in nature. Humans can make all but nine of them. The remaining nine are called essential amino acids and they must be supplied from what a person eats. If these amino acids are missing, then the person cannot manufacture the hundreds of proteins which are essential for its survival. Now it doesn't really matter how a person gets all twenty two amino acids. It's only important that he gets them. Most animal proteins are complete, which means they contain the nine missing amino acids, but there is a difference when we come to vegetable protein. Plant proteins usually are deficient in one or more essential amino acids, so to get complete proteins a variety of plants must be eaten. It makes good sense to eat less meat. But once you decide to substitute plant protein for animal protein, you must ensure that you get the complete set of amino acids regularly.

If you are not eating meat or dairy during a meal, you should have complementary carbohydrates. Meat complements any carbohydrate, so if meat is eaten at the meal even in small amounts, it will make up for the amino acids missing in the plants. Soybeans as a source of protein is as complete as animal protein, and it can be substituted for meat and dairy without any anxiety. But most others lack something and must be used with other plant protein to make up the complete complement of twenty two amino acids. As a rule of thumb, you can get the twenty two amino acids you need by combining any mature legume such as tofu, beans, and peanuts with whole grains such as wheat, rice, barley, oats or seeds; sunflower, pumpkin, etc.

Protein should account for 10-15% of your daily calories according to the RDA. Your main source of calories, 55-70% should come from complex carbohydrates. For some years complex carbohydrates have gotten a bad reputation. They are thought of as being starchy foods which the poor must live on, and which makes them fat. This is simply not the case. It is not the potato which makes a person fat. It is the butter or sour cream used to garnish it which is the big source of calories and which has little nutritional value. The potato, pasta, whole grain bread, and beans are rich sources of nutrients. The potato is a nutritional gold mine; it supples 5% of the day's supply of protein, 5% iron, 8% phosphorus, 10% thiamine, 11% niacin, and a whopping 50% vitamin C (if you eat it with the skin) a person needs per day. Complex carbohydrates are the major source of fiber in our diet (fiber comes from substances which make up the cell walls of plants). Although fiber is non nutritive, it is an essential dietary ingredient.

Carbohydrates are the physical body's main source of fuel. The problem is that in our affluence we consume too many processed foods which are high in refined sugars, high in calories and low in fiber and nutrients. Our insatiable sweet tooth cannot be gratified indefinitely without risk. With the average American consuming one third of a pound of sugar each day, the risk in terms of good health has become quite high. Let me preface our look at sugar with a little known fact: provided with enough starch to provide energy, a person needs no sugar in his diet at all. The problem with sugar is that it provides empty calories, calories with no nutritional value, and we simply don't need extra calories. We already know about the negative effect empty calories have on obesity and longevity, but there is also strong evidence which suggests that a high sugar diet may promote diabetes in people who are predisposed to it. There is really no case for having excess sugar and especially processed sugar in your diet.

The third major nutrient is fat. We get fat from both animal and vegetable sources. The vegetable sources are usually more benign, and are believed to be more easily digested and less of a health risk than animal fat. Fat is a more concentrated source of calories than any other nutrient and it is estimated that more than 40% of our calories come from fat. This is not a nutritionally healthy situation. Both complex carbohydrates and proteins provide calorie for calorie, much higher percentages of other essential nutrients, vitamins and minerals. Fat has more than twice the calories than either protein or carbohydrates per gram. Fats and especially animal fats are linked to life threatening diseases, such as heart disease, obesity, and cancer of the colon, breast and uterus. Obesity in itself is a risk factor in other diseases such as diabetes, obesity and liver disease. In addition, extra fat in the diet is harmful because in combination with other foods it causes digestion to be very slow and results in a sluggish metabolism, and cells receive nourishment slowly or not at all.

An interesting piece of research comes from the Dept. of the Navy, which supports the links between fat and disease; in 1977 the Navy studied the link between diet and expecially fat intake, with physical health and well-being. In the study the Navy compared the records of service men who had served in Vietnam, with servicemen who had been captured and served more than five years in Vietnamese prison camps. Their findings showed the servicemen who had been prisoners were on the whole more physically healthy than the control group. The Navy attributed their good health to the low fat, low cholesterol diet of rice, vegetables and occasional fish provided by their captors. There was no alcohol, coffee, and very little tobacco in their diet, plus their daily regimen included a program of vigorous physical exercise. [72]

Exercise and Health
Exercise is another essential part of a daily regimen of

good health. Exercise can be anything from walking to the corner, cleaning the house, to mountain climbing or wind-surfing. There are physical activities which fit every lifestyle and which, when done regularly and in appropriate amounts, add to your well-being and good health. Let's remember human beings evolved as hunters and gatherers, and in more primitive times people performed all sorts of strenuous physical activity on a daily basis. Physical activity was not only necessary for survival, but the activity required to survive also kept the physical body operating at peak performance. Jane Brody tells us, "Exercise is the best way I know for getting something for nothing (or next to nothing). It is an all around tonic for body and mind. The physical and psychological benefits of exercise could go a long way toward reducing the need for medical care and improving the quality of life—your life, whether you're eight, eighteen, forty eight, or eighty eight."[73] Jane Brody is not alone in her endorsement of exercise. In 1700 John Dryden penned these verses:

> Better to hunt in fields, for health unbought,
> Than fee the doctor for a nauseous draught.
> The wise, for cure, on exercise depend;
> God never made his work for man to mend."[74]

Modern researchers have found that regular exercise offers a host of health benefits unknown in earlier times. The latest evidence indicates that regular exercise reduces the risks of heart attack. It improves the distribution of oxygen throughout the body tissue, which in turn increases a person's capacity for work. People who perform vigorous physical activity regularly are found to have lower cholesterol levels than more sedentary people, and physical conditioning improves the blood's ability to remove clots which could cause obstructions in the heart, lungs or brain. As an added benefit, regular exercise can be an important tool in treating diabetes. Lack of exercise on the other hand leads to a loss of calcium in the bones, and this increases their susceptibility to fracture, and as a person gets older the chances are increased for developing osteoporosis, the loss of bone with age. Among the other benefits of regular exercise are an enhanced sense of well-being, better muscle tone, healthier skin, better concentration and a better self-image.

Being Healthy Everyday

Any regimen designed to promote and maintain good health must take a human being's complex nature into consideration. It must promote balance and harmony on all four planes; must keep the subtle energy system healthy and must promote positive attitudes and relationships. To begin you must put away those things in your environment which have a negative impact on your health. They could be anything from self-doubt and negative relationships to hazardous chemicals. It might help to make a list of the things which you think have a negative influence on your life and contribute to disease. Then stop worrying about them, and instead begin transmuting negative thinking through positive programming. Use the techniques you learned to change negative thoughts into positive ones. Then pick out those things you could change with little or no effort and make a commitment to do so immediately. Next, pick out those things which would be hard to change and begin reprogramming using affirmation and visualization. Finally, for those things you can't change, find a way to change your relationship to them. For example, if you drive to work and you are continually caught in traffic jams, which drive you to distraction, distract yourself by installing a tape deck and learning a new language. Avoid lumping stressful events and stressful people together, but spread them out and budget your time so you can be rid of them as quickly as possible. Pay attention to your body and slow down when it gives you warning signals such as back aches and headaches. In addition, find time to do the things that reduce stress in you life and make you feel good. Even if you only have a few minutes, you can practice Yogic breathing, or you can go to your sanctuary.

But the best health insurance is you. Be consistent. Start each day with chakra balancing and let it take you into a short meditation. Twenty to thirty minutes is enough to start the day right, and if you pay attention after your meditation, you will find that staying in the alpha state afterwards is easy. Use part of your meditation for affirmations and visualizations; use one segment for short term problem solving, and another segment for long term reprogramming. Spend the remaining time in your sanctuary. Then have a hearty and nutritious breakfast. Try to make breakfast the biggest meal of the day. If you have free time between breakfast and lunch, then practice mental projection. If you are walking between appointments, try the exercise below. I call it the walking Yogic breath. As you walk, inhale deeply for four steps (taking a deep Yogic breath) and exhale deeply for four steps. Keep breathing in this rhythm, without separation between inhalation and exhalation, until you enter the alpha level. Then combine affirmations with the Yogic breath and reprogram while you walk. You could begin on an inhalation by affirming, "Healing energy is flowing into me," and then on the exhalation, "healing me on all levels". You can use different affirmations, depending on how you feel. Lunch should be your second largest meal, and you should try to eat it at the same time each day. Remember that regularity at meal times cues the body clocks and keeps them rhythmic. Try to take some time to relax after you've eaten. Take a siesta and do something that makes you feel good.

Daily exercise is an important part of a daily regimen of good health. So, take every opportunity to exercise. Start a weekly workout schedule. To stay in peak condition you should exercise vigorously (work up a sweat) at least three times a week. However, for those of you who haven't done strenuous exercise in some time, or for those of you who are over forty, begin by seeing a doctor and be sure to take a stress test. A stress test will tell you the condition of your cardio-vascular system. Always begin an exercise program slowly, and always warm up before and after you exercise. Consult a fitness expert before you embark on a comprehensive exercise program, or pick up one of the books available on the subject. They will give you hints on what to do and what not to do.

The time between work and dinner is a perfect time to unwind and do a long healing meditation. Try to put aisde one hour before dinner for meditation and healing. During your meditation, work on long term goals by using affirmations and visualization, and practice your breathing exercises. Practice the techniques of absentee healing, and end by going to your sanctuary for some private time alone. Remember, by healing others you will be healing yourself. If you are wound up at the end of the work day because of pressure on the job, or because the kids are driving you crazy, begin your evening meditation with chakra balancing or with the bellows breath. Either technique will bring you back into the alpha state. The evening meditation is a perfect time for the family to get together, so try to arrange a family meditation. You will benefit immeasurably from meditating and healing together. Not only will it bring you closer together, it will make your meditations and healings more profound because of the dynamics of the group. Dinner should be the smallest meal of the day. Remember to give your body the chemical rest it needs after dinner. Try to put aside one day of the week as a fast day. Avoid stimulants and get the rest you need each night by getting sufficient sleep. Your evening activities are up to you. I would only caution you that excessive and addictive activities are antithetical to health. Strive always to stay in balance, and as my teacher often told me, "Pay attention; remember who you are and be thankful."

SOURCE NOTES

1. Shri P. Swami, (trans. by) *The Geeta, The Gospel of the Lord Shri Krishna*, London, Eng.: Faber and Faber, 1935, p. 73.
2. Rabindranath Tagore, *Songs of Kabir*, New York, N.Y.: Samuel Wieser, Inc., 1915, p. 23.
3. C. I. Scofield, ed., *Holy Bible, King James Version*, New York, N.Y.: Oxford University Press, Heb. 5:6.
4. Three Initiates, *The Kybalion: Hermetic Philosophy,*. Chicago, Il.: Yoga Pub. Soc., 1912, p. 26.
5. Ibid., p. 28.
6. Ibid., p. 30.
7. Ibid., p. 32.
8. Ibid., p. 35.
9. Hippocrates, *Breaths, Book One.*
10. *The Kybalion*, p. 38.
11. *Holy Bible*, Gal. 5:7.
12. *The Kybalion*, p. 39.
13. *Holy Bible*, Isaiah 6:13-14.
14. Ibid., II Timothy 1:7.
15. Vatiswarananda, *Adventure in Religious Life*, Madras, India, 1959, p. 263.
16. Dr. Carl O. and Stephanie Simonton, *Attitudes of the Cancer Patient*, Laredo, Texas: Silva Mind Control International, Inc.
17. *Holy Bible*, II Kings 4:17-23, 32-36.
18. Sheila Ostrander and Lynn Schroeder, *Superlearning*, New York, N.Y.: Dell Publishing Co., 1979, p. 3.
19. *Holy Bible*, Matt. 17-20.
20. *The Geeta*, p. 38.
21. *The Kybalion*, p. 28.
22. Alice Bailey, *Esoteric Healing*, New York, N.Y.: Lucis Publishing Co., 1953, p. 83.
23. Hugh Lynn Cayce, *The Edgar Cayce Reader No. 2*, New York, N.Y.: Warner Books. 1969, p. 121.
24. *Holy Bible*, John 1:1-3.
25. *Holy Bible*, Luke 18:17.

202   *The Art of Spiritual Healing*

26. D. C. Lau, (trans. by) *Tao Te Ching*, New York, N.Y.: Penguin Books, XLVII, vs. 107, 1963, p. 108.
27. P. D. Ouspensky, *The Fourth Way*, New York, N.Y.: Random House Inc., 1959, p. 8.
28. *Holy Bible*, Heb. 11:1.
29. Ibid., Heb. 11:6.
30. *Edgar Cayce Reader No. 2*, p. 62.
31. *Holy Bible*, Prov. 22:24-25.
32. *The Kybalion*, p. 43.
33. Emile Coue, *Self Mastery Through Conscious Auto-Suggestion*, Boston, Ma.: Allen and Unwin Inc., 1922.
34. Lawrence Cherry, "The Power of the Empty Pill", *Science Digest*, Vol 89, No. 8, 1981, p. 116.
35. *Esoteric Healing*, p. 141-142.
36. *Holy Bible*, John 7:38.
37. *Holy Bible*, Rom. 5:5.
38. *The Kybalion*, p. 43.
39. Chitrita Devi. *Upanisads For All*, Ram Nagar, New Delhi, India: S. Chand and Co. Ltd., 1973, Kathopanisad 14, p. 40.
40. Yogi Ramacharaka, *Science of Breath,* Chicago, Il.: Yogi Publication Society, 1904, p. 28.
41. Eugen Herrigel, *Zen in the Art of Archery*, New York, N.Y.: Vintage Books, 1953, p. vi.
42. *Holy Bible*, Jer. 33:3.
43. *The Geeta*.
44. Carl and Stephanie Simonton, James Creighton, *Getting Well Again*, New York, N.Y.: Bantam Books, 1978, p. 8.
45. S. G. J. Ouseley, *The Power of the Rays*, Mokelumne Hill, Ca.: Health Research, 1957, p. 24.
46. S. G. J. Ouseley, *The Science of the Aura*, Romford, Essex, Eng.: L. N. Fowler and Co. Ltd., 1949, p. 22.
47. Edna St. Vincent Millay, *Collected Lyrics:"Renascence"* New York, N.Y.: Harper and Row, 1917.
48. *Upanisads For All*, Svetasvataropanisad, vs. 11-13, p. 121-122.
49. *Holy Bible*, Eph. 2:10.

50. Campbell Holms, *The Facts of Psychic Science and Philosophy*, New Hyde Park, N.Y.: University Books Inc., 1969, p. 478.
51. *Holy Bible*, James 5:16.
52. Ibid., John 9: 1-7.
53. Ibid., Mark 5: 35-30.
54. *Breaths, Book One.*
55. *Edgar Cayce Reader No. 2*, p. 67.
56. Possiduis, *Life of St. Augustine*, 29 in Deffa, Early Christian Biography, 1952, p. 111.
57. *The Kybalion*, p. 30.
58. *Holy Bible*, Rom. 5:5.
59. *Holy Bible*, John 7:38.
60. *The Kybalion*, p. 39.
61. *Holy Bible*, Matt. 6:22.
62. *Upanisads For All*, Svetasvataropanisad vs. 7, p. 99.
63. Edward Taylor, *The Reflection: The Mentor Book of Major American Poets*, New York, N.Y.: Mentor Books, p. 43.
64. Gay Luce, *Biological Rhythm in Human and Animal Psychology*, New York, N.Y.: Dover Publications, p. 10.
65. Ibid., p. 11.
66. Roy Walford, *Maximum Lifespan*, New York, N.Y.: Avon Books, p. 100.
67. Ibid., p. 103.
68. Dr. Henry Bieler, *Food Is Your Best Medicine*, New York, N.Y.: Ballantine Books, p. 18.
69. Karen MacNeil, *Whole Foods*, New York, N.Y.: Vintage Books, p. 22.
70. *Food Is Your Best Medicine*, p. 27.
71. Jane Brody, *New York Times Guide To Personal Health*, New York, N.Y.: Avon Books, p. 1.
72. *Whole Foods*, p. 33.
73. *New York Times Guide To Personal Health*, p. 85.
74. John Dryden, *Epistle to John Dryden of Chesterton*, line 92.

INDEX

STAY IN TOUCH

On the following pages you will find some of the books now available on related subjects. Your book dealer stocks most of these and will stock new titles in the Llewellyn series as they become available. We urge your patronage.

To obtain our full catalog, to keep informed about new titles as they are released and to benefit from informative articles and helpful news, you are invited to write for our bimonthly news magazine/catalog, *Llewellyn's New Worlds of Mind and Spirit*. A sample copy is free, and it will continue coming to you at no cost as long as you are an active mail customer. Or you may subscribe for just $10.00 in the U.S.A. and Canada ($20.00 overseas, first class mail). Many bookstores also have *New Worlds* available to their customers. Ask for it.

Llewellyn's New Worlds of Mind and Spirit
P.O. Box 64383-720, St. Paul, MN 55164-0383, U.S.A.
* * *

TO ORDER BOOKS AND TAPES

If your book dealer does not have the books described, you may order them directly from the publisher by sending full price in U.S. funds, plus $3.00 for postage and handling for orders *under* $10.00; $4.00 for orders *over* $10.00. There are no postage and handling charges for orders over $50.00. Postage and handling rates are subject to change. We ship UPS whenever possible. Delivery guaranteed. Provide your street address as UPS does not deliver to P.O. Boxes. Allow 4-6 weeks for delivery. UPS to Canada requires a $50.00 minimum order. Orders outside the U.S.A. and Canada: Airmail—add retail price of book; add $5.00 for each non-book item (tapes, etc.); add $1.00 per item for surface mail.

FOR GROUP STUDY AND PURCHASE

Because there is a great deal of interest in group discussion and study of the subject matter of this book, we offer a special quantity price to group leaders or agents. Our special quantity price for a minimum order of five copies of *The Art of Spiritual Healing* is $23.85 cash-with-order. This price includes postage and handling within the United States. Minnesota residents must add 6.5% sales tax. For additional quantities, please order in multiples of five. For Canadian and foreign orders, add postage and handling charges as above. Credit card (VISA, MasterCard, American Express) orders are accepted. Charge card orders only ($15.00 minimum order) may be phoned in free within the U.S.A. or Canada by dialing 1-800-THE-MOON. For customer service, call 1-612-291-1970. Mail orders to:

LLEWELLYN PUBLICATIONS
P.O. Box 64383-720, St. Paul, MN 55164-0383, U.S.A.

Prices subject to change without notice.

THE INNER WORLD OF FITNESS
by Melita Denning

Because the artificialities and the daily hassles of routine living tend to turn our attention from the real values, *The Inner World of Fitness* leads us back by means of those natural factors in life which remain to us: air, water, sunlight, the food we eat, the world of nature, meditations, sexual love and the power of our wishes—so that through these things we can re-link ourselves in awareness to the great non-material forces of life and of being which underline them.

The unity and interaction of inner and outer, keeping body and psyche open to the great currents of life and of the natural forces, is seen as the essential secret of *youthfulness* and hence of radiant fitness. Regardless of our physical age, so long as we are within the flow of these great currents, we have the vital quality of youthfulness: but if we begin to close off or turn away from those contacts, in the same measure we begin to lose youthfulness. Also included is a metaphysical examination of AIDS.

This book will help you to experience the total energy of abundant health.

0-87542-165-2, 240 pgs., 5¼ x 8, illus., softcover   **$7.95**

CHAKRA THERAPY
by Keith Sherwood

Keith Sherwood presents another excellent how-to book on healing. His previous book, *The Art of Spiritual Healing* has helped many people learn how to heal themselves and others.

Chakra Therapy follows in the same direction: Understand yourself, know how your body and mind function and learn how to overcome negative programming so that you can become a free, healthy, self-fulfilled human being.

This book fills in the missing pieces of the human anatomy system left out by orthodox psychological models. It serves as a superb workbook. Within its pages are exercises and techniques designed to increase your level of energy, to transmute unhealthy frequencies of energy into healthy ones, to bring you back into balance and harmony with your self, your loved ones and the multidimensional world you live in. Finally, it will help bring you back into union with the universal field of energy and consciousness.

Chakra Therapy will teach you how to heal yourself by healing your energy system because it is actually energy in its myriad forms which determines a person's physical health, emotional health, mental health and level of consciousness.

0-87542-721-9, 270 pgs., 5¼ x 8, illus., softcover   **$7.95**

THE LLEWELLYN PRACTICAL GUIDE
TO CREATIVE VISUALIZATION
by Denning & Phillips

All things you will ever want must have their start in your mind. The average person uses very little of the full creative power that is his, potentially. It's like the power locked in the atom—it's all there, but you have to learn to release it and apply it constructively.

IF YOU CAN SEE IT. . . in your Mind's Eye . . . you will have it! It's true: you can have whatever you want—but there are "laws" to mental creation that must be followed. The power of the mind is not limited to, nor limited by, the material world—Creative Visualization enables Man to reach beyond, into the invisible world of Astral and Spiritual Forces. Some people apply this innate power without actually knowing what they are doing, and achieve great success and happiness; most people, however, use this same power, again unknowingly, incorrectly, and experience bad luck, failure, or at best an unfulfilled life.

This book changes that. Through an easy series of step-by-step, progressive exercises, your mind is applied to bring desire into realization! Wealth, power, success, happiness even psychic powers . . . even what we call magickal power and spiritual attainment . . . all can be yours. You can easily develop this completely natural power, and correctly apply it. Illustrated with unique, "puts-you-into-the-picture" visualization aids.
0-87542-183-0, 294 pgs., 5-1/4 x 8, illus., softcover   **$8.95**

THE LLEWELLYN PRACTICAL GUIDE TO ASTRAL PROJECTION
by Denning & Phillips

Is there life after death? Are we forever shackled by time and space? The ability to go forth by means of the Astral Body, or Body of Light, gives the personal assurance of consciousness (and life) beyond the limitations of the physical body. No other answer to these ageless questions is as meaningful as experienced reality.

The reader is led through the essential stages for the inner growth and development that will culminate in fully conscious projection and return. Not only are the requisite practices set forth in step-by-step procedures, augmented with photographs and "puts-you-in-the-picture" visualization aids, but the vital reasons for undertaking them are clearly explained. Beyond this, the great benefits from the various practices themselves are demonstrated in renewed physical and emotional health, mental discipline, spiritual attainment, and the development of extra faculties.

Guidance is also given to the Astral World itself: what to expect, what can be done—including the ecstatic experience of Astral Sex between two people who project together into this higher world where true union is consummated free of the barriers of physical bodies.
0-87542-181-4, 266 pgs., 5-1/4 x 8, illus., softcover   **$8.95**

KUNDALINI AND THE CHAKRAS
A Practical Manual—Evolution in this Lifetime
by Genevieve Paulson

The mysteries of Kundalini revealed! We all possess the powerful evolutionary force of Kundalini that can open us to genius states, psychic powers and cosmic consciousness. As the energies of the Aquarian Age intensify, more and more people are experiencing the "big release" spontaneously but have been ill-equipped to channel its force in a productive manner. This book shows you how to release Kundalini gradually and safely, and is your guide to sating the strange, new appetites which result when life-in-process "blows open" your body's many energy centers.

The section on chakras brings new understanding to these "dials" on our life machine (body). It is the most comprehensive information available for cleansing and developing the chakras and their energies. Read *Kundalini and the Chakras* and prepare to make a quantum leap in your spiritual growth!

0-87542-592-5, 224 pgs. 6 x 9, illus., color plates   **$12.95**

HOW TO SEE AND READ THE AURA
by Ted Andrews

Everyone has an aura—the three-dimensional, shape-and-color-changing energy field that surrounds all matter. And anyone can learn to see and experience the aura more effectively. There is nothing magical about the process. It simply involves a little understanding, time, practice and perseverance.

Do some people make you feel drained? Do you find some rooms more comfortable and enjoyable to be in? Have you ever been able to sense the presence of other people before you actually heard or saw them? If so, you have experienced another person's aura. In this practical, easy-to-read manual, you receive a variety of exercises to practice alone and with partners to build your skills in aura reading and interpretation. Also, you will learn to balance your aura each day to keep it vibrant and strong so others cannot drain your vital force.

Learning to see the aura not only breaks down old barriers—it also increases sensitivity. As we develop the ability to see and feel the more subtle aspects of life, our intuition unfolds and increases, and the childlike joy and wonder of life returns.

0-87542-013-3, 160 pgs., mass market, illus.   **$3.95**

PRACTICAL COLOR MAGICK
by Raymond Buckland

The world is a rainbow of color, a symphony of vibration. We have left the Newtonian idea of the world as being made of large mechanical units, and now know it as a strange chaos of vibrations ordered by our senses, but our senses are limited and designed by Nature to give us access to only those vibratory emanations we need for survival. But we live far from the natural world now. And the colors which filled our habitats when we were natural creatures have given way to gray and black and synthetic colors of limited wavelengths determined not by our physiological needs but by economic constraints.

Learn the secret meanings of color. Use color to change the energy centers of your body. Heal yourself and others through light radiation. Discover the hidden aspects of your personality through color.This book will teach all the powers of light and more. You'll learn new forms of expression of your innermost self, new ways of relating to others with the secret languages of light and color. Put true color back into your life with the rich spectrum of ideas and practical magical formulas from *Practical Color Magick!*

0-87542-047-6, 136 pgs., illus., softcover $6.95

THE WOMEN'S BOOK OF HEALING
by Diane Stein

At the front of the women's spirituality movement with her previous books, Diane Stein now helps women (and men) reclaim their natural right to be healers. Included are exercises which can help YOU to become a healer! Learn about the uses of color, vibration, crystals and gems for healing. Learn about the auric energy field and the Chakras.

The book teaches alternative healing theory and techniques and combines them with crystal and gemstone healing, laying on of stones, psychic healing, laying on of hands, chakra work and aura work, and color therapy. It teaches beginning theory in the aura, chakras, colors, creative visualization, meditation, health theory and ethics with some quantum theory. Forty-six gemstones plus clear quartz crystals are discussed in detail, arranged by chakras and colors.

The Women's Book of Healing is a book designed to teach basic healing (Part I) and healing with crystals and gemstones (Part II). Part I discusses the aura and four bodies; the chakras; basic healing skills of creative visualization, meditation and color work; psychic healing; and laying on of hands. Part II begins with a chapter on clear quartz crystal, then enters gemstone work with introductory gemstone material. The remainder of the book discusses, in chakra by chakra format, specific gemstones for healing work, their properties and uses.

0-87542-759-6, 352 pgs., 6 x 9, illus., softcover $12.95

WHEELS OF LIFE AUDIO CASSETTE
by Anodea Judith
Here is the ultimate listening experience. A journey through the sounds and sensations of the chakras created by Anodea Judith especially for Llewellyn and you! With guided meditations, powerful poetry, and original music composed and performed by Bay Area keyboardist/producer Rick Hamouvis, Wheels of Life will entertain and enlighten in the tradition of the best Llewellyn has to offer. If you are reading this book, you must have the tape!
0-87542-321-3   **$9.95**

WHEELS OF LIFE: A User's Guide to the Chakra System
by Anodea Judith
An instruction manual for owning and operating the inner gears that run the machinery of our lives. Written in a practical, down-to-earth style, this fully-illustrated book will take the reader on a journey through aspects of consciousness, from the bodily instincts of survival to the processing of deep thoughts.

Discover this ancient metaphysical system under the new light of popular Western metaphors—quantum physics, elemental magick, Kabbalah, physical exercises, poetic meditations, and visionary art. Learn how to open these centers in yourself, and see how the chakras shed light on the present world crises we face today. And learn what you can do about it!

This book will be a vital resource for: Magicians, Witches, Pagans, Mystics, Yoga Practitioners, Martial Arts people, Psychologists, Medical people, and all those who are concerned with holistic growth techniques.

The modern picture of the Chakras was introduced to the West largely in the context of Hatha and Kundalini Yoga and through the Theosophical writings of Leadbeater and Besant. But the Chakra system is equally innate to Western Magick: all psychic development, spiritual growth, and practical attainment is fully dependent upon the opening of the Chakras!
0-87542-320-5, 544 pgs., 6 x 9, illus., softcover   **$14.95**

THE HEALER'S MANUAL
A Beginner's Guide to Vibrational Therapies
Ted Andrews

Did you know that a certain Mozart symphony can ease digestion problems ... that swelling often indicates being stuck in outworn patterns ... that breathing pink is good for skin conditions and loneliness? Most dis-ease stems from a metaphysical base. While we are constantly being exposed to viruses and bacteria, it is our unbalanced or blocked emotions, attitudes and thoughts that deplete our natural physical energies and make us more susceptible to "catching a cold" or manifesting some other physical problem.

Healing, as approached in *The Healer's Manual,* involves locating and removing energy blockages wherever they occur—physical or otherwise. This book is an easy guide to simple vibrational healing therapies that anyone can learn to apply to restore homeostasis to their body's energy system. By employing sound, color, fragrance, etheric touch and flower/gem elixers, you can participate actively within the healing of your body and the opening of higher perceptions. You will discover that you can heal more aspects of your life than you ever thought possible.

0-87542-007-9, 256 pgs., 6 x 9, illus., softcover $10.00